▪ HOW NATURAL REMEDIES WORK ▪

D0701400

How Natural Remedies Work

&

BY

JO SERRENTINO

Hartley & Marks, *Publishers*

Published in the U.S.A. by
Hartley & Marks, Inc.
Box 147, Point Roberts
Washington
98281

Published in Canada by
Hartley & Marks, Ltd.,
3663 West Broadway
Vancouver, B.C.
V6R 2B8

Printed in the U.S.A.

Text © 1991 by Jo Serrentino

All rights reserved.
Except for brief reviews, no part of this book may be
reproduced in any form or by any means, electronic or mechanical, including
photocopying, recording, or by any information storage and retrieval system, without
the written permission
of the publisher.

ISBN 0-88179-030-3

Typeset by The Typeworks in Meridien
Cover design by Elizabeth Watson
Chapter opening graphics by Marian Bantjes

If not available at your local bookstore,
this book may be ordered from the publisher.
Send the cover price plus one dollar
fifty for shipping to either of the
above addresses.

LIBRARY OF CONGRESS CATALOGING-IN-PUBLICATION DATA
Serrentino, Jo, 1957-
How natural remedies work : vitamins, minerals, nutrients,
homeopathic, and naturopathic remedies : how to choose them, how
they are manufactured, how they prevent and heal illness / Jo
Serrentino.
p. cm.
Includes bibliographical references and index.
ISBN 0-88179-030-3 (pbk.) : $11.95 ($14.95 Can.)
1. Herbs--Therapeutic use. 2. Therapeutics, Physiological.
I. Title
RM666.H33S47   1991
615.5'8--dc20 91-20090   CIP

*This book is dedicated with love to my husband Robert
and to two very special beings in my life,
Racket the dog and Hardley the cat.*

■ ■ ■

> *The ideas, methods, and suggestions in this book are not intended as a substitute for consultation with a physician.*

I am grateful to Dr. Harlan Lahti, pharmacist, for his role as consultant. I wish to thank all those researchers who too often go without credit for their very important part in providing pieces to the scientific puzzle. My gratitude to all those at Hartley & Marks who participated in the creation of this book and made it a truly enjoyable project.

Contents

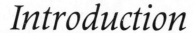

Introduction

The prevention and treatment of illness with natural substances has come a long way in the last decade. It has moved from an alternative way of life to a science.

In today's world filled with synthetics, pollutants, and contaminants, more people are finding comfort in natural substances, organic foods, and biological medicines. What used to appeal to those practicing an alternative lifestyle now attracts people from all walks of life.

But the natural-health industry is having difficulty communicating factual information. Regulations introduced by such government agencies as the Food and Drug Administration in the United States and Health and Welfare in Canada prevent the inclusion of technical information on product labels.

This effort to protect the consumer actually confuses matters by protecting products that are poorly manufactured and not subjected to the rigorous quality controls essential to the production of natural remedies. This book provides information so that you can recognize good and bad natural remedies. All natural remedies are not created equal! Manufacturing processes make a great deal of difference in the effectiveness of a natural remedy. Natural remedies carry the properties of their sources. In addition to the therapeutic properties of the plant source, extracted substances produce biochemical frequencies that affect the energy patterns of the body, realigning body systems to vibrate with improved health. Certain methods of extraction and manufacturing destroy both these energies and many active therapeutic substances, rendering the remedy ineffective and even, in some cases, deleterious. Once you have a basic understanding of natural substances, you will better be able to choose effective natural remedies.

This book also explains what you should look for in different types of remedies. It describes the effectiveness of different types of remedies and reveals how their properties can be altered during manufacturing. Explanations of scientific procedures and examples of scientific research provide scientific evidence of the effectiveness of natural remedies.

Unlike pharmaceutical drugs, natural remedies address every system of the body. In this sense, they are holistic. Holism considers every aspect of an illness and treats the whole being, rather than the symptoms alone, as orthodox allopathic medicine often does. Historical records as far back as 400 B.C. reveal this split between the allopathic and holistic medical approaches. This book explores the reasoning behind both approaches, explaining natural remedies and the holistic approach in scientific terms.

Already, as our perspective of medicine changes, we can see that the battle between allopathic and holistic ways and remedies is subsiding. More and more allopathic practitioners are turning to holistic approaches. This book attempts to merge the two disciplines with a new perspective. By applying scientific reasoning and examples of research to natural remedies, this book shows how such remedies work. And by describing the effectiveness of natural remedies and holistic treatments, as observed clinically, perhaps this book will lead to a greater appreciation of new age medicine. After all, is it not a fact of science that two opposite forces can merge to form a whole greater than each part?

ONE

The Bioenergetics and Manufacture of Natural Remedies

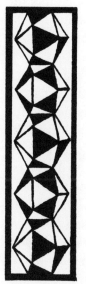

Bioenergetics is the branch of biology dealing with the energy frequencies of all living systems. In every biosystem energy flows, and this total energy is made up of the energy frequencies of individual ills. But labels on natural remedies are often misleading, because the biological and therapeutic properties of ingredients cannot be listed unless the product has a DIN—drug identification number. With a DIN, medical claims can be made; however, laws in Canada prevent the inclusion of many claims, even on products that have DINS. U.S. laws are much more liberal, and more information is allowed on labels. But no natural-product labels in the United States or Canada may reveal the therapeutic use of the product. You will notice that health-product labels never state what a product is for. This is because information about what the product is for and how it works must be approved by the Food and Drug Administration (FDA) to be included in the label. However, the FDA's trend is to approve only medical research. Politics often prevents funding for research on preventive health products and subsequent approval by the FDA. Even when medical research is carried out on health products, and the studies published in medical journals, the findings are not allowed to be mentioned by their manufacturers or sellers. It is hoped that the growing interest of the major pharmaceutical companies in natural products will spur new label regulations that will allow more information to be included on packaging.

Essential oils illustrate the difference that can exist between product types. An essential oil is a pure, fragrant liquid extracted from a plant. The chemical composition and, subsequently, the therapeutic applications of an essential oil vary according to the species of plant used for extraction. The laws governing information on labels prohibit the listing of indications and do not require that the source plant be specified. Thus, essential oil of sage may come from garden sage *(Salvia officinalis)*, or from sclarated sage *(Salvia sclaria)*. *Although the essential oils from both species may smell the same to the untrained nose, their chemical makeup is entirely different.* *Salvia officinalis* yields an essential oil with a high content of ketones (a chemical group), which have anticoagulant, sedative, and mucinolytic (mucus-thinning) properties. *Salvia sclaria* yields an essential oil with a high content of esters (another chemical group), which have mainly antispasmodic effects. Since essential oil of sage is sold as the essential oil extracted from *Salvia officinalis* whether it is extracted from this species or not, you cannot be sure of the properties of the specific essential oil you are buying.

To further complicate matters, the chemical composition of essential oils also depends on where the plant was grown, growth conditions, life stage of the plant, and when it was harvested. In addition, manufacturers using plants from areas where soil may be contaminated, or wild varieties that have not been analyzed for their specific chemical composition, can get away with selling their essential oil as the standard. Finally, products made from poor-quality ingredients or from raw materials that have not been tested for quality are often touted to be as therapeutic as those that are properly manufactured under stringent conditions. These factors are the main reasons why rigorous quality controls are essential to the production of natural remedies.

Many companies develop ineffective products because of the source materials they use to make their formulae. At raw-materials auctions, many manufacturers buy the cheapest ingredient, not the one with the best quality and consistency. Other companies copy established remedies, using questionable raw materials that may not have the active principles required to yield the therapeutic properties the formula should possess. Still other companies farm out the contract to manufacture their remedy, eliminating any control over the consistency of the product. These delinquent procedures contribute to the doubt associated with natural remedies and may lead to dangerous substitutes.

THE ENERGY PATTERN OF THE BODY'S CELLS

The body starts to heal at the cellular level. The state of cells depends on their surroundings, and just as changes in the environment affect the lower creatures in the ecosystem first, the disease state attacks at the cellular level first. The body's cells are grouped into organs and the organs into systems. To be effective, the active ingredients of a remedy must reach the cells of the body. For a remedy to act at the cellular level, it must have the right energy pattern.

Every living thing has energy. Our body's cells are bathed in energy fields that receive information from their surroundings and transmit the digested information back into their surroundings. The energy field of each cell is part of a network that connects organs and systems throughout the body, forming a life-sustaining bioenergy circuit. This intricate circuitry underlies all healing of the body and health. The interaction of the energy patterns of cells, organs, and systems contribute to growth and repair of all of the biosystems in the body.

The substances that we ingest, whether they are food, drugs, or natural remedies, all have their own energy pattern. That is, the molecules that make up these remedies have a certain structure that gives them a specific energy pattern. For our body's cells to perform their tasks and keep the body functioning normally, they need to interact with substances that possess a compatible energy pattern. We can compare the process to the running of a car—we use gasoline, not alcohol or water, to fuel a car. The car's performance depends on the type of gas used (whether it is high octane, leaded, or unleaded). The car's emissions also depend on the gas used. Similarly, for biochemical interaction to occur at the cellular level, there must be compatibility both between substances and between substances and "machinery" (in this case, the body or biosystem).

BIOENERGETICS OF THE BODY

The Meridian System

Chinese medicine, which has been thriving for over 2,000 years, works with an energy principle called the meridian system. This principle includes the idea that acupuncture points, or acupoints, exist along an invisible meridian system that runs throughout the tissues of the body. In 1967 this system was studied in Korea by Professor Kim Bong Han. He injected a radioactive isotope into a rabbit's acupoint and followed the pathway of the isotope as it was absorbed by surrounding tissue. He discovered that the isotope was being taken up a minute tubular system whose path corresponded to the acupuncture meridians.

French researcher Pierre de Vernejoul's experiments substantiated these findings in humans by injecting a radioactive isotope into the acupoints of human subjects and recording the pathway through gamma-radiation imaging. It was confirmed that the isotope travelled along classical Chinese acupoints and that the meridians formed a system separate from other channels in the body, such as those in the venous or lymphatic system. A cardinal energy flows along this invisible meridian, nurturing all body structures. The Chinese call this cardinal energy, "chi." According to traditional Chinese medical doctrine, in a healthy body the chi must flow normally without interruption.

Medical studies carried out in Korea and in Europe confirmed the existence of the acupuncture meridian pathway. Further testimony that energy flows through an invisible meridian system is provided by the recent development of several diagnostic devices. The first is the Motoyama AMI machine, which makes use of electrical information from acupuncture points. Electrodes are attached to the body at defined acupoints on the main meridians. Traditional Chinese medicine proposes twelve pairs of meridians that connect specific biosystems within the human body. The AMI machine compares the electrical balance between the right and left sides of the body, and its computer analyzes the electrical differences. The principle of the AMI machine is based on the Chinese principle of yin and yang, which states that the internal organs of a healthy body have paired meridians of identical and balanced electrical energy. *Energy flows through organs via paired meridians on the left and right sides of the body. When illness is present or pending, this energy flows unevenly through the paired meridians.* On the AMI machine, this uneven flow registers as an electrical imbalance between the two sides of the body. By discovering electrically unbalanced acupoints, the AMI machine can identify existing or potential problem areas within the meridian-associated biosystems. Stated another way, the AMI machine can measure the energy fields of cells and biosystems.

Another diagnostic system that works in a similar fashion is the Voll machine (sometimes called the Dermatron). The Voll machine, invented by a German physician of that name, differs from the AMI machine in that it can measure the electrical field at any acupoint on the body. In addition to identifying which organs have unbalanced energy, the Voll machine can detail the dysfunction of the organ. The Voll machine also has a metallic platform that holds vials of any remedy to be tested. In this way, the energy pattern of the remedy becomes part of the energy circuit of the Voll machine. Skilled practitioners using the Voll machine can test several remedies by observing the electrical changes that occur in the body's acupoints. They can determine if the electrical frequencies are matched, and if the remedy has an energy pattern that is compatible with that of the patient's body.

Resonance

The principle behind matching frequencies and energy patterns with such diagnostic machinery as the Voll machine is a biophysical phenomenon known as resonance. To understand this phenomenon, it is necessary to describe our bodies at a cellular level. The smallest component of matter is the atom. Constituents of the atom that carry an electrical charge are called electrons. Electrons circle the center of the atom (the nucleus) in energy levels or shells, and within these shells, in orbitals. For an electron to move from a lower level to a higher level of energy, a certain amount and specific pattern of energy is required. The atomic frequency required to move an electron from one level to another is called the resonant frequency or free oscillation frequency.

It is difficult to drive a system at any frequency other than its free oscillation frequency. Thus, remedies can only drive the biosystem to "vibrate"—or heal—if they have a compatible energy pattern.

The active principles in a remedy must have a compatible energy pattern with that of the cells of the human body. When in a state of illness, the human body oscillates at a different frequency from when it is healthy. A gentle push with the appropriate energy frequency in the needed energy pattern will cause the natural healthy oscillating frequency to return by realigning the energy patterns of different biosystems. Natural remedies contain the subtle energy frequencies needed to push the body to its healthy energy pattern.

Active Principles

Active principles are ingredients extracted from a plant that have therapeutic properties. These might be decongestant, sedative, or analgesic properties, for example. However, many manufacturing processes destroy these active principles, leaving the remedy without any therapeutic value. Other processes may damage an ingredient by altering its cellular structure. This in turn alters the energy pattern of the active principle, making it incompatible with the energy pattern of the body's cells. Breaking down a natural substance into its active principles alters its energy. As you have seen, each element of a biosystem possesses an energy pattern that contributes to a collective energy pattern. Although the active principles of plants contain the therapeutic properties, other elements within the biosystem also contribute to the energy patterns. These changes in therapeutic effectiveness are discussed in more detail in a later chapter.

THE BIOCHEMICAL RELATIONSHIP OF A REMEDY WITH THE BODY

All of the body's cells are surrounded by chemicals. These chemicals relay information to the entire biosystem by passing through channels in the cell membranes and carrying on intricate biochemical reactions. Just as the body has an energy balance, it also has a chemical balance. Just as cells and their energy pattern are affected by their immediate surroundings, so the biochemical condition of the body is affected by outside forces—specifically, by what gets into our bodies through the foods we eat, the drugs we take, and even the infiltration of environmental pollutants. Chemical and energetic harmony within the body contributes to wellness. The use of natural remedies supports the balance of processes and the harmony between biosystems within the body.

A physical law, the second law of thermodynamics, applies to the way biological remedies work in the body: As an energy-conversion process, such as cellular respiration, progresses, the cell's entropy (disorder) decreases; but as individual cellular reactions occur, entropy of the biosystem (the body) increases.

Our body is a machine that runs on biochemical reactions. It is programmed to handle all incoming substances (such as drugs and food) through biochemical reactions, to transform them, absorb them, and eliminate residues. The body processes everything. We don't have to push any buttons or program the processes; we fuel the body and it eliminates the rest. But since the second law of thermodynamics tells us that as more processes occur in a machine, the more they contribute to disorder and to the subsequent loss of energy of the machine, *we should pay some attention to the quality of substances we put into our body "machine."* We should choose substances that do not contribute to disorder—pure, energetically compatible substances that break down efficiently without unnecessary biochemical reaction.

When you use natural remedies, you are fuelling your body with compatible energy. In a sense, you are inserting the right key. If the energy pattern of the substance you are using is compatible with your body, it will not have to go through extra biochemical reactions leading to entropy. Don't forget that your body is a biochemical factory, and it will use whatever substance you put into it—whether good or bad—in a biochemical reaction. The more biochemical reactions that occur, the more disordered the biosystem will become.

Biological substances that are fully compatible with the constituents of the biosystem actually will help to maintain a balance. They create a smooth-running machine that uses its energy to make you feel good and enjoy life. Synthetic substances always leave toxins in the body. Since energy is required for all processes, energy is also required to rid the body of toxins left by synthetic substances. This elimination process involves more biochemical reactions, leading to entropy, or disorder.

THE DIFFERENCE BETWEEN ALLOPATHIC AND NATURAL REMEDIES

Just as the cells of the body gain information from and react to their surroundings, the active principles in herbs or flowers have their own energy pattern or electrical field. When we isolate active principles, we are plucking them from their "natural" surroundings, changing the energy pattern that gives them direction, and consequently altering their action. Of course, the active element alone will contribute a fundamental frequency and action, but the harmony that exists in the whole compound will be lost.

Lecithin, a substance that contains the nitrogen and phosphorous found in the tissue of living things and that is marketed as a nutritional supplement, has been the subject of a number of scientific experiments. The active principle of interest in lecithin is phosphatidyl choline. Choline, one of the B complex vitamins, is necessary in fat metabolism in plants and animals. It is involved in many biochemical reactions, mainly as a precursor of enzyme reactions. Enzymes are proteins that catalyze biochemical reactions. They hook onto molecules, causing them to be transformed. One study used choline to treat a movement disorder, tardive dyskinesia, which is a side effect of certain drug therapies. The experiment found that isolated choline acted in half the time it took lecithin (the whole complex containing choline), but the reaction of lecithin lasted three times longer than that of pure choline. Moreover, fewer side effects were associated with lecithin. Lecithin contains a lot of fat that must be removed or lecithin granules will become rancid. For this reason, many manufacturers bleach or deodorize lecithin. It has been discovered that these processes destroy the valuable choline content of lecithin.

These findings seem to suggest that a natural balance is being transferred from one living system to another. The use of non-processed, natural ingredients reinforces healing by contributing compatible energy, and the intermingling of active principles with other ingredients within the biosystem somehow acts to regulate the body's biochemical balance.

Conventional allopathic drugs have a certain kind of action in the body, which reverses itself after a specific time—usually about two weeks. At this point they induce the body's biochemistry to oppose the action of the drugs. In pharmaceutical terms, this is known as the biphasic effect, meaning simply that a drug has two phases. In phase one, the drug acts on the body. In phase two, the body's biochemistry counteracts the drug. For example, an antihistamine will stop the production of histamine, a local hormone that causes, among other symptoms, swelling and the stimulation of nerve endings that causes pain and itching—two symptoms often associated with allergies. The antihistamine drugs will stop the allergylike symptoms by blocking receptors—molecules in a cell membrane that produce a temporary compound (like histamine), which change the cell's function. Antihistamine drugs provoke a kind of competition with the body's histamine for the receptor that would naturally take up histamine.

In other words, antihistamine drugs will provide you with temporary relief but will stimulate your body to produce more histamine (and discomfort) in the long run. This biphasic action of allopathic drugs shows us that *allopathic drugs do not heal the body but rather biochemically block the substances causing the symptoms.* This action throws the body's biochemistry off balance, causing more biochemical reactions and leading to greater disorder. This constant compensation taxes the body, tending to keep it in a state of illness. In this sense, allopathic drugs are cumulative. They do not realign the body's biochemistry, producing a cure, but cause the body to expend energy to fight foreign substances.

ENERGY PATTERNS OF ALLOPATHIC VERSUS NATURAL REMEDIES

Active principles extracted from natural substances do not have a problematic cumulative effect on the body. Energy is transferred from one living system to another, and this energy gives molecules direction and a certain action. The body's cells receive information from their surroundings. Scientists demonstrated this when they took cultured cancer cells and returned them to a healthy body. The cells regained "healthy" direction from their healthy surroundings and began to react in a balanced biochemical fashion. The molecules of active principles taken from natural substances contain this "healthy" data, received from the markers or memory banks of the cells in their healthy living systems. Even when the active principles are no longer part of the whole, they will retain this information. Often, they do not react as they would when they are part of the whole (as with lecithin). However, if they are properly extracted from an organic, living source, they will possess the energy and action they had when they were part of the whole.

Synthetic drugs do not have markers, because they are artificially formulated; they are not extracted from living systems. They do not contribute an energy pattern, because they never existed as a biosystem. The only thing they contribute is the biphasic effect. *Instead of providing a channel for the body to realign its energy pattern, synthetic substances alter the natural rhythm of the body, bringing it further out of balance and into entropy.*

WHAT IS NATURAL?

The terms "natural," "organic," and "biological" are often lumped together, when in fact each term has a separate meaning. The term "natural" is most often used collectively to describe organic, biological, and naturally occurring substances. More specifically, it refers to a substance that exists naturally, that does not have to be produced synthetically, but that may not be pure. According to the food industry, sugar is a natural substance. The term "natural" most often suggests a product containing some naturally occurring substances that are refined, or processed without organic methods, or that contain additives or chemical preservatives. A good example of such a product is aloe vera. *Many aloe products contain pure aloe vera gel, but they also contain synthetic preservatives that may cause skin allergies or irritations.* This type of formulation undermines the value of aloe vera and causes confusion about the effectiveness of pure products.

WHAT IS ORGANIC?

When a product or a substance is labelled organic, it is understood that all of the substances it contains are derived from elements grown in unpolluted soil, without the use of herbicides, insecticides, fertilizers, or fungicides. Soil and water samples are taken at regular intervals set by the independent organic grower. These samples are analyzed in the laboratory to determine if they contain any toxic elements, chemical by-products, or radioactive materials that may have infiltrated the soil or water bed from the surrounding environment. In Europe, products are analyzed for levels of toxic materials by independent laboratories that have been appointed by the government of the country. The product must receive an LMR (Limite maximale des résidus nocifs). This is the certified maximum amount of toxic residues a product may contain and still be sold. The standards or allowed amounts of toxic materials are established by the government of each European country. *No official standards determining toxic residues exist in the United States or Canada.* Neither government enforces any kind of policy for organic growers. The Food and Drug Administration (FDA) of the United States government enforces labeling laws and establishes the amount of ingredients a product may contain (especially for vitamins and minerals). In Canada, Health and Welfare enforces the same regulations. However, these have nothing to do with whether a product or its ingredients are organic.

Organic substances are thought to be more compatible with our bodies than nonorganic substances. The reason for this may be in the energy pattern of a substance. Since the energy pattern of an organic substance is derived from living elements, its energy pattern is closer to that of the cells of the living body, giving the organic substance greater compatibility with the body. Greater compatibility means that the body's cells are better able to absorb the substance and that an organic remedy will be more effective than a nonorganic remedy.

WHAT IS BIOLOGICAL?

A biological product is composed of organic elements that yield an energy pattern compatible with the cells of the body and make the product biologically active. To say that a product is "biologically active" means that the frequency between the molecules of the components of the remedy and that of the components of the body are compatible. A biologically active product acts somewhat like a key that fits the molecules within the body's cells. If the product's molecules fit into the body's molecules, the product will be much more active than products composed of nonorganic elements.

To manufacturers, the terms "biological," "organic," and "natural" are buzz words that are often used loosely to mislead the unsuspecting consumer. This is unfortunate, and though natural remedies are better adapted to the body than synthetic drugs, they are often misrepresented, either through ignorance or deliberate marketing strategies.

People are often skeptical about natural remedies, and one sometimes hears statements like, "It's just a herb—it's not strong enough." Many an overdose or toxicity has occurred because of this attitude. The motto "If a little is good, a lot is better" does not apply to biological remedies, because they are very concentrated. These substances are organic chemicals, a pure form of the active component and the most potent form. Pharmaceutical preparations are usually made with inorganic chemicals, although the pharmaceutical industry does manufacture natural remedies using elements taken from nature; some may have been organically grown, but most come from nonorganic sources. The molecular structure of a pharmaceutically natural formula is based on the organic structure of the naturally occurring model substances. But since manufacturing a molecule chemically is usually less expensive than extracting and stabilizing active principles from a plant source, the synthetics are the most widely sold substances.

ESSENTIAL OILS AND TINCTURES

Essential oils are a good example of therapeutically active biological substances. *The essential oils produced by a plant are components of the plant's immune system.* An essential oil is composed of several different organic chemical groups, and thus a synthetically derived molecule of an essential oil can be "constructed" using inorganic molecules from the same chemical groups extracted from nonorganic products. An essential oil made by nature and extracted from a plant, however, is more potent than a synthetically manufactured essential oil. Often it is up to ten times more concentrated. And the properties of the naturally derived essential oil are more specific than those of its inorganic, synthetically derived counterpart.

The same is true of the energy level of tinctures. Tinctures are remedies made from dilutions of plant extracts. Plants grown either organically or inorganically are separated into parts—leaves, stems, roots, flowers—chopped, and soaked in alcohol for about 10 days. This process is called maceration. The macerated plants are then pressed, and the extract is collected. The extract may be in the form of a liquid—from plants that yield a liquid when pressed—or in the form of a paste—from plants that yield little liquid. In either form, the extract contains the active principles of the plants. The solubility of these active principles will determine the concentration of alcohol in the tincture, which can vary from 10 percent to 50 percent. Alcohol is the preferred solvent in manufacturing tinctures since it dissolves the active principles of the extract and keeps them stable without altering the energy of their molecules.

One will rarely find an undiluted plant extract for sale as a remedy, because most extracts are so strong that they are difficult to dose safely. A pure plant extract can be found as a tincture or as a hydrolysate. A hydrolysate, which is a by-product of extraction, consists mostly of water and only a small concentration of extract. It is used in the same way as a tincture and is rarely cheaper, even though it is a much weaker solution. A plant extract must always be capsulized or suspended in an alcohol solution to remain stable and effective.

VITAMINS AND MINERALS

The importance to health of vitamins and minerals is widely accepted today. The rumor of their benefits began with body builders and quickly spread to the general public. Today vitamin and mineral therapy has proven itself. Vitamins are known as necessary nutrients that our bodies cannot manufacture. Although they are recognized as essential to our body's biochemical processes, it is still widely believed that if one has a nutritionally balanced diet, there is no need for vitamin and mineral supplementation. Although our bodies can extract vitamins from food, large quantities of specific food sources are required to extract the necessary amounts of vitamins—about a pound of wheat germ for every 50 international units (IUS) of vitamin E, or four pounds of rice for every 50 milligrams of a B vitamin. Vitamin and mineral supplements are much more convenient.

Minerals—often called trace elements because they are not

required by the body in large quantities—are believed to be more effective in a chelated form. A chelated mineral is one that has been chemically bound to an amino acid. Amino acids belong to a class of organic acids that occur in all plant tissue and in animal tissue. They are considered the building blocks of protein. In the body, a mineral will naturally bind to an amino acid. The amino acid acts as a transporter for the mineral, allowing it to be properly assimilated by the body instead of being carried right through the digestive tract unused. Since a chelated mineral is a mineral already bound to an amino acid, it has a built-in transporter. Although as yet no scientific evidence exists showing that the chelated form of a mineral is better than the nonchelated form, such a process may make a difference in the efficacy and therapeutic properties of mineral supplements.

Not all available vitamin and mineral supplements are created equal. Because of the current interest in vitamin therapy, research in nutritional supplementation is growing. As a result, new formulae have evolved and are being produced, and we must become aware of the differences between them. *The value of a "natural" product, and how efficiently it works in the body, depends on the product's engineering and purity.*

The chart below lists the manufacturing process for each type of product described in this book, including the pages where the process is described in detail. The chart also suggests what textures to look for, including the pages where these features are described in detail.

PRODUCT	MANUFACTURING PROCESS	WHAT TO LOOK FOR
minerals	chelation (p:tk)	mineral complexes (p:tk)
tonics: yeast-based or plant extracts	plasmolysis (p:tk)	organic production (p:tk)
essential oils	vapor distillation	label stating that they are guaranteed 100% pure

PRODUCT	MANUFACTURING PROCESS	WHAT TO LOOK FOR
	(p:tk)	and biologically certified (p:tk)
vitamins	pure crystallization (p:tk)	organic sources (p:tk)
amino acids	peptide bonding (p:tk)	
herbs in capsules	lyophilization (p:tk)	freeze-drying (lyophilizing) (p:tk)

FOR FURTHER READING

Baerlein, E. and Dower, A. *Healing with Radionics: The Science of Healing Energy.* Wellingborough, England: Thorsons Publishers, 1980.

Barbeau, A.; Growdon, J. E.; and Whurtman, R. J. *Nutrition and the Brain.* New York: Raven Press, 1979.

Black, Dean. *Health at the Crossroads.* Springville, Utah: Tapestry Press, 1988.

Curtis, Helena. *Biology.* New York: Worth Publishers, 1975.

Gelenberg, A. J., et al. "Choline and Lecithin in the Treatment of Tardive Dyskinesia: Preliminary Results from a Pilot Study." *American Journal of Psychiatry* 136 (June 1979).

Gerber, Richard. *Vibrational Medicine.* New Mexico: Bear & Co., 1988.

Growdon, S. H., et al. "Normal Plasma Choline Responses to Ingested Lecithin." *Neurology* 30 (1980).

Haber, D. A., et al. "Properties of an Altered Dihydrofolate Reductase Encoded by Amplified Genes in Cultured Mouse Fibroblasts." *Journal of Biological Chemistry* 256 (September 1981).

Porcellati, G.; Amaducci, C.; and Gallo, C. *Function and Metabolism of Phospholipids.* New York: Plenum Press, 1976.

Robertson, M. "Nerves, Molecules and Embryos." *Nature* 278 (April 26, 1979).

Rubin, H. "Cancer As a Dynamic Developmental Disorder." *Cancer Research* 45 (July 1985).

Sirotnak, F. M., et al. "Relative Frequency and Kinetic Properties of Transport Defective Phenotypes Among Methotrexate-resistant

L1210 Cell Lines Derived *in vivo.*" *Cancer Research* 41 (November 1981).

Tansley, D. *Radionics and the Subtle Anatomy of Man.* Essex, England: Health Science Press, 1972.

"Tracking a Molecule's Progress." *Science News* 133 (February 13, 1988).

Wurtman, R. J., et al. "Lecithin Consumption Raises Serum-free Choline Levels." *Lancet* (July 9, 1977).

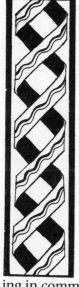

TWO

Holism

The term "holism" conjures up images of antiquated medical techniques that have nothing in common with science and technology. Some people think that holism appeals to those seeking an alternative lifestyle and to those who are opposed to allopathic medicine. In fact, this is not only a dim view of holism but also an erroneous one.

LOOKING AT THE WHOLE PERSON

The holistic approach is far removed from kettles and jars of strange herbs and magic rituals. As the word implies, holism means to look at the whole—holism is often spelled "wholism." When holism is applied to illness, it looks at all the circumstances associated with an illness, considering the body and the person as a whole.

Holistic medicine is not practiced only by alternative-health professionals, like naturopaths and homeopaths. Many doctors originally trained in allopathic medicine have adopted the holistic approach, realizing that it is a thorough and natural way to treat the body.

As discussed in chapter 1, allopathic medicine often treats only symptoms, and allopathic drugs have a two-phase effect that causes the body to fight back, resulting in a vicious circle that keeps the body in a state of repair rather than well-being. Often the ends justify the means; because allopathic drugs provide quick relief of symptoms, people do not question their long-term effects on the body. The fast results are demanding on the body and often cause other problems that will be treated in the same manner. In contrast, *holism reviews a person's collective symptoms, the condition of the body, and the patient's circumstances, lifestyle, and environment. The objective of the holistic approach is to strengthen the body, inducing a healthful state.* Allopathic medicine strives to relieve symptoms by introducing compounds it thinks the body requires. But the continual manipulation of the body's biochemistry by allopathic methods keeps the body in a state of disorder and disease. Allopathic medicine has a relatively small repertoire of remedies, which relieve symptoms or reduce or increase a substance the body is producing (like a hormone). In addition to causing stress to the body, this small repertoire reduces the body's healing abilities. In contrast, holistic practitioners are more likely to use any method that has been shown to work. Holism is not really a branch of medicine, nor should it be confused with a philosophy. Rather it is an approach to a problem that does not impose the stringent guidelines used in allopathic medicine. Unfortunately, this open-mindedness has given holism a reputation as a practice based on vague philosophies.

Holism asks why the patient has a medical problem. The diagnosis consists of a physiological and emotional investigation, with the intent of awakening the patient's self-awareness. Since a major objective of holism is to determine the source of the medical problem, there is a thorough exchange of information between physician and patient. Not only are specific physical causes addressed, as in allopathic medicine, but all possible links to the illness are investigated. For example, stress can be a cause of a physical illness. Prescribing an allopathic drug will not remove the stress; instead, it will place physical stress on the body, causing the problem to persist and often to become worse. (Stress-related illness is discussed in chapter 10.)

With physical illness, it makes sense to investigate the patient's emotions as well. This holistic principle is based on biological evidence that cells gain information from their surroundings. *Since cells get information from their surroundings, causing them to change their energy patterns and action, disturbed emotions can also sabotage the body.* After all, emotions are a part of the "whole" biosystem of the human being. Holistic practitioners have reported how their patients alleviated such ailments as constipation or nervous asthma by verbalizing pent-up feelings. In addition, a decision to get well may be enough to trigger the body's healing powers. Since the allopathic approach does not view the system as a whole, it does not explore other avenues that might be causing a medical problem. It simply looks at one part of the system—the part that has the damage.

Of course not all disorders are linked to lifestyle or external forces (from the surrounding environment). Many, such as genetic disorders, are aberrations of a physiological system. But it has been clinically observed that *all* conditions respond to treatment of the whole system. Making a system stronger inevitably diminishes an attacking force.

Properly practiced, holism is an excellent approach to illness that can enhance allopathic medicine. Natural remedies apply particularly well to holistic medicine because they offer the same kind of adjuvant reinforcing or enhancing treatment. Most biological remedies contain many plant extracts to treat a whole condition rather than just a symptom. *For instance, to treat flu, a naturopath or homeopath may use a herbal extract that contains seven plant extracts.* One plant extract may thin mucous secretions, one may be a decongestant for all of the breathing passages, one may be an anti-inflammatory for neuralgia associated with flu, one plant extract or homeopathic ingredient may help reduce fever, one may suppress cough, one may help the body relax so that it can heal, and often one might be a tonic or supplement to help the body maintain strength while it is spending all its energy to heal. Compare this with common over-the-counter allopathic remedies, which may be fever-reducing medicines, analgesics, or cough suppressants. The most complete over-the-counter cold medicine combines an antihistamine with vitamin C.

EVALUATING SYMPTOMS

To compare the holistic approach with the allopathic from the point of view of symptoms, let's say that you have the following complaints: itchy, runny eyes, sneezing, fatigue, sore muscles and joints, headache, loss of appetite, coughing, and possibly fever. One might suppose that these are cold symptoms. But what about allergy or food intolerance? The symptoms are the same. Looking at the overall picture, a physician might ask: Have you eaten anything different? Have you felt like this before? Have you been exposed to people with cold or grippe? The answers may give a diagnosis that is significantly different. In fact, these symptoms can even be caused by hormones and warn of the onset of menstruation in women.

Evaluating only the symptoms to diagnose a condition and to choose a remedy is not necessarily effective. A holistic approach studies the condition as a whole, then uses the following procedures:
– Physiological testing—running allopathic tests, like blood tests, X rays, and urine analysis. If possible, tests that may induce stress and thus heighten or trigger symptoms are avoided.
– Psychological testing—evaluating the present condition of the patient, measuring stress, and investigating any psychosomatic connections to the patient's physical condition.
– Lifestyle evaluation—evaluating the amount of stress associated with lifestyle and reviewing diet, pace of life, and exercise.

PRESCRIBING A PROGRAM

The holistic approach often uses allopathic testing procedures and evaluations for both physiological analysis and psychological analysis. The results of these tests are then examined by qualified physicians, and a whole program, rather than just a remedy, is prescribed. A holistic program may involve the following components:

−Biological remedies
−Nutritional supplements
−Dietary changes
−Exercise techniques or relaxation techniques or a combination of both
−Mental exercise
−Spiritual exercise

Biological remedies contain ingredients that zero in on the organ or area of the body that is causing the symptoms. They do not mask the symptoms but treat the underlying condition by causing the body to begin repairing its altered state. This process will alleviate the symptoms as well. Allopathic medicine often masks the symptoms without treating the condition.

Nutritional supplements provide a source of extra energy that the body needs when it is healing itself. Illness often suppresses the appetite, so the body does not get the nutrients it needs to perform all the biochemical reactions that go on during healing. Thus, supplements are an important adjuvant to any remedy.

Diet is an important factor in health at all times but particularly during healing. When the body is in repair, it works overtime. If one eats foods that are difficult to digest, the body must work even harder. It must spend energy to break down the food, depleting the fuel supply already in the body and the fuel that the food is supplying. The same depletion of energy occurs if one eats food that is poor in nutrients, because the body must spend energy to digest food that will not refuel it. The body is spending the energy it badly needs for healing and is not getting any energy in return. If one eats food that contains a lot of preservatives and chemicals, the body's energy will be seriously depleted, and toxicity of the system will be increased, because of the many biochemical reactions that occur during healing. These biochemical reactions have by-products that must be eliminated. If the food ingested leaves residues, energy will be required to eliminate them also. And illness itself saturates the body with toxins that require energy to be eliminated. Thus, diet directly affects the state of an illness and the recovery time of an individual.

Exercise helps eliminate toxins. But too much exercise may cause overoxygenation of the body. When the body oxygenates, it fills its cells, tissues, and organs with oxygen. Too much oxygen can cause undesirable biochemical reactions that produce such toxins as lactic acid. Lactic acid causes the characteristic cramping and pain in muscles that professional athletes, especially runners, sometimes experience. One's normal exercise program usually has to be adapted to the altered energy pattern that occurs during illness.

Certain types of exercise provide both physical toning and mental relaxation and are unparalleled for health and healing. An excellent example of such an exercise is a Chinese exercise method called tai chi chuan. This type of "soft exercise," as it is sometimes called, is regarded as a body/mind exercise because both the body and the mind are trained during the practice. Prescribed by health practitioners in both allopathic and holistic medicine, soft exercise has been found to be beneficial in the treatment of chronic diseases as well as in psychosomatic illness. Tai chi chuan provides harmony between body and mind by helping to realign the body's energy pattern and maintaining the flow of the body's cardinal energy, or chi.

Mental exercise is often overlooked during illness, especially by allopathic medicine. The best example is how we treat our children during illness. Usually they are kept in bed, and all normal activity ceases. Although under certain conditions it is impossible to concentrate, at some stage even in serious illnesses work can be resumed on a partial schedule. *Without mental stimulation, illness gains power over one's attitude and psyche. This phenomenon may produce other physical ailments and cause mental sickness that will make it much more difficult for the patient to heal.*

Spiritual exercise is also necessary to human nature. Most people believe in something, someone, or some way of life. Illness tends to dull our spiritual nature, especially at the onset of a serious illness. Healing is slowed when one's spiritual side is depressed. It is important to keep spirituality intact, for it plays an invaluable role in the healing process.

USING HOLISTIC REMEDIES

Holistic medicine does not put stress on the body as allopathic medicine can. Often the introduction of drugs used in allopathic medicine to mask symptoms upsets the body's components or biochemistry. This altered condition is usually manifested as side effects. For instance, tranquilizers, so often recommended by allopathic medicine to treat the stress-induced ailments of modern life, can cause drowsiness, confusion, depression, loss of memory, dizziness, blurred or double vision, headaches, and liver damage.

The breakdown of pharmacological drugs in our bodies can result in biochemical reactions whose by-products destroy cells and tissues. Or drugs can accumulate in the body and bind with enzymes, preventing them from performing vital metabolic functions. Other drugs can depress the immune system, making the body more vulnerable to illness, infection, stress, and disease.

Nonactive ingredients called excipients, used as fillers, coatings, or binders in the manufacture of drugs, are extraneous and must be eliminated by the body. Digestion of these excipients may cause stomach upset, as do analgesics.

Holistic remedies treat the body as a whole with natural, noncumulative substances that strengthen the body rather than tax it. Holistic remedies do not simply provide relief; they attempt to heal the condition.

Take the example of menstrual discomfort. Allopathic medicine tends to treat menstrual discomfort with analgesics. Some of the recommended analgesics are over-the-counter pain remedies, whereas others require prescription. After the patient is examined for physiological causes of her pain, the allopathic approach will recommend these types of remedies. Allopathic medicine will rarely consider nutrition and lifestyle, which can both cause upsets in the menstrual cycle by changing the chemical balance of the brain.

A study conducted at the Massachusetts Institute of Technology indicates how carbohydrate consumption can influence mood by changing the chemical processes within the brain, causing symptoms associated with premenstrual syndrome (PMS)—a condition that occurs before menstruation, causing mood swings, depression, water retention, tender breasts, nausea, headaches, and cravings (usually for sugar).

The holistic approach to menstrual discomfort investigates the physical condition of the patient to see whether the pain is caused by an inflammation due to infection, polyps, or other physical causes. But it also explores the patient's diet, lifestyle, and psychological state. Moreover, the holistic approach tries to resolve the entire problem rather than treating only the pain, exploring all avenues connected with menstrual physiology and the menstrual cycle. For instance, pain can be caused by excess swelling due to water retention or to poor circulation, which can be treated nutritionally. In fact, studies indicate that the use of certain amino acid combinations can alleviate menstrual problems by re-establishing the biochemical balance of the menstrual cycle—the source of the problem.

The menstrual cycle starts in the brain at the hypothalamus, a gland that controls other glands in the body; it is the master switch. The brain is essentially a pharmacy that uses chemicals produced from the breakdown of the foods we eat. These chemicals stimulate certain processes in the brain that control the physiological functions of the body. The resulting rise and fall in the concentration of hormones that triggers the hypothalamus and pituitary to become active is a process called negative feedback. When this process is unbalanced, menstrual problems can occur. Pain is only one of the symptoms that may stem from a hormonal imbalance.

Allopathic medicine usually treats such a hormonal imbalance with oral hormones, which cause the body to fight back, provoking a loss of natural rhythm. Moreover, hormones are known to cause many side effects, such as excessive hair growth. In contrast, holistic medicine uses a homeopathic remedy that contains a natural substance to intercept the menstrual cycle. This remedy causes more hormones (or fewer hormones, depending on the problem) to be naturally released by the body, rather than saturating the body with oral hormones and shocking it into drastic cyclical changes, which in turn cause other problems and side effects.

ALLOPATHIC AND HOLISTIC MEDICINE

It is unfortunate that many scientists and allopathic doctors can find scientific relevance only in the test tube. It is even more unfortunate that they do not understand that their test-tube findings, restricted by their controlled environment, do not reflect the complexities of an open biosystem—like the human body—that is influenced by all kinds of outside factors that cannot be accounted for in a laboratory experiment. Microbiologist René Dubos eloquently discusses this point in his book *Man Adapting*. In 1965, he predicted that medicine would wallow in "a sea of irrelevancy" unless it paid more attention to the relationship between the body system and its total environment.

Holism looks at the person's harmony with his or her environment, whereas allopathic medicine tends to look at a single cause, not the whole picture. The body is a self-contained system, with a natural rhythm. Allopathic medicine—except in life-and-death situations that require surgical intervention—interferes with the body's natural flow. Randomly, and for a time, allopathic drugs help the system, but they do not change (energize) or reorganize or harmonize the system as organic substances can with their energy. Allopathic drugs are synthetic, and the body cannot readily assimilate them, further reducing the body's ability to find natural rhythm. In this sense, allopathic medicine is working against the biosystem's nature. It is well known that every time humans have gone against nature, they have suffered dire consequences.

Holism involves our whole environment. It does not arbitrarily control the patient but rather allows him or her to participate in the healing process, and to influence the body's healing mechanisms. This participation is in itself a healing process for the patient. A person, animal, or plant that is nurtured responds; a person, animal, or plant that is restrained fights back. *The more humane approach of holism offers a freedom that allows a person to feel in control. And feeling in control of one's life and body is a state of health.*

ASKING THE RIGHT QUESTIONS

When you go to a health professional for treatment, you are putting your health in his or her hands. Below are questions you can ask to help you choose the right professional and the best approach to your illness.

Finding Out about the Treatment

What questions should I ask my doctor or health professional?

1. Does the treatment you are prescribing cause any unpleasant side effects or dependency?
2. What happens if I don't follow the treatment?
3. What happens if I don't complete the treatment and the medication?
4. Will this treatment get rid of this condition permanently?
5. Will I have to repeat this treatment?
6. Is this treatment demanding on my body, or will it strengthen my body?
7. How long will this treatment last?
8. When can I expect to start feeling results?
9. What can I expect from this treatment?

Finding Out about Medications or Remedies

What questions should I ask my druggist or health-remedy representative?

1. What will this medication do?
2. How does this medication work inside my body?
3. Does this medication cause any unpleasant side effects or dependency?
4. Are there any excipients that are dangerous to the metabolism in this medication?
5. Is this medication specific to one area of the body, and to my condition, or does it affect other unrelated parts of my body?
6. Are there any foods or drinks or drugs I should avoid while taking this medication?
7. Can I go out in the sun while I am on this medication? Can

I take it if I'm pregnant?
8. Should I take this medication on an empty or a full stomach?
9. Are there any activities I should refrain from doing while taking this medication?
10. How long is the recommended treatment period for this medication and when can I expect to start feeling results?
11. Exactly what is this remedy made of?

FOR FURTHER READING

Wurtman, R., and Wurtman, J. "Carbohydrates and Depression." *Scientific American* (January 1989).

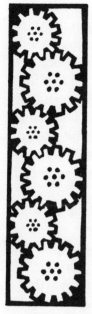

THREE

Manufacturing Techniques

The efficiency, digestibility, and efficacy of a natural remedy is directly related to the way it is manufactured. There may be vast differences in health products containing the same ingredients, depending on the type of process used to form the mixture.

THE IMPORTANCE OF RAW MATERIALS

The source of the raw materials, which in natural remedies are mostly herbs, plant extracts, and other biological substances, is the most important factor in determining the quality of a product. Most companies that have their products manufactured by independent laboratories give up quality control of raw materials. Companies that manufacture products in-house, however, preserve control over their raw materials; even if they do not grow or produce the raw materials, they test each batch of raw materials for purity and for the amount of active principle it contains. This batch-testing of raw materials is known as a bioassay. More sophisticated and expensive testing is done with chromatographic machines that determine the active ingredients of a particular substance by generating bands of color on a photographic plate. Each colored band represents an active ingredient. This procedure is called a chromatographic analysis and is the "fingerprint" of the substance. An incident occurred within the North American industry several years ago that illustrates the importance of controlling the quality of raw materials. *An independent laboratory decided to test most of the oil of evening primrose on the market. The results were astounding: out of all the products tested, only one contained gamma linoleic acid—the active principle of oil of evening primrose.* The lack of proper manufacturing controls contributed to this delinquency.

The analysis of raw materials to determine their complete composition, either in active principles or in contaminants and radioactive substances, is crucial, but because it is a time-consuming and expensive step, most manufacturers do not batch-test raw materials. The consumer cannot tell whether a product has been batch-tested or not. Often labels include claims such as "organically produced," which ensures only that the raw materials are organic. Other labels state that their product has been analyzed or bio-assayed; this practice is rare, but it ensures purity. One way to get to the root of the matter is to ask your retailer—he or she should know. If the retailer does not know, then he or she can find out. If your retailer cannot find this information for you, you should probably shop elsewhere. Such retailers are not committed to and may not even believe in their products and do not trust in their quality.

Where else can you get health products? If you live in a small town that does not have a health-food store or where there is only one, there are alternatives.

—Ask your local drugstore or convenience store to order products for you. Give them the product package so that they can trace the distributor.

—Check your yellow pages for health-product representatives that service your area.

—Order by mail through national health magazines.

MANUFACTURING PROCESSES

The health-remedies industry chiefly uses processes that have been proven effective. Although new products are marketed every year, most new products are produced by old methods. This chapter reviews processes that over the years have produced effective remedies.

Each type of product has a characteristic manufacturing process. For example, plasmolysis is a procedure involving yeast, which applies to yeast-based supplements, tonics, and certain extracts. Certain manufacturing processes make a difference in the effectiveness of the product. In Europe, a study in which over one thousand allopathic doctors used plasmolyzed yeast products to treat patients suffering from general fatigue with lack of concentration and mood swings showed a marked improvement in these patients, compared with those using ordinary yeast tonic that had not been plasmolyzed. The study indicated that the plasmolyzed yeast tonic significantly changed four aspects of illness—mood, fatigue, appetite, and sleep—areas that are commonly disturbed in most illnesses.

Similarly, studies comparing chelated minerals with nonchelated minerals reveal that chelated minerals reduce the time required for the body to metabolize the mineral and therefore do not deplete the body of energy that can be used in performance. X rays of the colon of healthy college students showed that nonchelated minerals often passed through the digestive tract completely undigested.

Plasmolysis: A Process That Produces Tonics

Plasmolysis is a unique process involving the culture of yeast cells that is usually used to make tonics. Plasmolyzed yeast products differ from other yeast products in having a greater biological character and thus yielding potent tonics. Cultures of yeast cells, usually *Candida utilis*, are fed on fresh plant extracts.

The yeast is grown on a medium—usually a gelatinous substance called agar-agar—that contains plant extracts. As the yeast cells grow and divide, they incorporate the active principles of the plant extracts into their cells; they do this in the same way that the cells of the human body would assimilate these plants as food.

Once the yeast cultures are ready, plump with the active principles of the plants they have been feeding on, they are plasmolyzed—exploded—in order to release the contents of their cells. Next, the liquified cells are strained to remove the cell membranes. Final results yield a concentrated yeast solution containing the active components of the plant extracts used in the culture medium. In this form the solution is a highly available source of these plant substances. The body cells recognize the molecules and are able to assimilate them quickly. This natural assimilation occurs because the plasmolyzed yeast product is compatible with the body; it thus has great potency.

The active principles from the plant extracts have specific effects on the body's organs and functions. In addition, the plasmolyzed yeast solution provides the nutrients contained in yeast (see chart below).

The Active Principles in Yeast

AMINO ACIDS	VITAMINS	MINERALS
arginine	biotin	calcium
choline	vitamin C	cobalt
cystine	cobalamin	copper
glutamic acid	folic acid	iron
glutathione	inositol	magnesium
glycine	nicotinamide	manganese
histidine	pantothenic acid	phosphorus
isoleucine	pyridoxine	potassium
leucine	riboflavin	silica

AMINO ACIDS	VITAMINS	MINERALS
lysine	thiamine	sodium
methionine	nicotinamide	sulfur
phenylalanine	biotin	
threonine	pantothenic acid	
tryptophan	folic acid	
tyrosine	cobalamin	
valine	inositol	

Plasmolysis yields a solution ready for the body. The effects of plasmolyzed yeast preparations on the defense mechanism of the body have been well documented in several scientific studies throughout the world. Experiments by the European Space Agency, and by the National Aeronautics and Space Administration (NASA) in spacelab and the space shuttle, reveal that a plasmolyzed yeast tonic considerably increases the activity of lymphocytes, or defense cells. In contrast, ordinary yeast products simply mix several elements together to produce a formula, instead of using a process like plasmolysis to integrate all the elements into a new substance.

Best choice: physiologically and economically, plasmolyzed yeast solutions are a better value.

Vapor Distillation to Yield Essential Oils

Vapor distillation is an extraction process, usually used to extract essential oils. It is a simple process that involves the distillation of plant parts to yield an essential oil and a hydrolysate. A copper or stainless still that contains a separate chamber where the plant parts are placed is used. The separate chamber is an important factor because it ensures that the hot water will not touch the plant materials and thus will not break down or dilute the essential oils. Instead, the water vapor slowly extracts the essential oil from the plant materials.

The raw materials are as important in vapor distillation as they are in plasmolysis and many other manufacturing processes. However, vapor distillation emphasizes the time of harvest of the plants. The chemical makeup of an essential oil changes at different stages of a plant's life, and therefore the period of time between harvest and actual distillation is a prime factor in determining the therapeutic nature of an essential oil.

It is very difficult for consumers to know whether the essential oils they purchase are produced through vapor or water distillation. Fortunately, most essential oils are derived from vapor distillation. The important thing to look for on a label is the following phrase: "100% guaranteed pure and botanically certified."

European health products are analyzed and controlled for the presence of contaminants. In Europe, products derived from plants are analyzed for contaminants that may come from chemicals used on soil near growing crops, or from pollution. If any harmful contaminants are found, the batch is rejected and will not receive certification. Each European country that adheres to this regulation has its own standard that determines the concentration of contaminant that is acceptable for human consumption. Each batch of a product is analyzed by a designated laboratory assigned by the government of that country. Switzerland, Austria, Belgium, and Italy follow this practice. *In the United States and Canada, there are no government regulations forcing manufacturers to check the concentration of contaminants of their products.* Those manufacturers that stamp their products "certified biological" subscribe to the European analysis of testing for contaminants, usually setting higher standards and performing the analysis in their own laboratories at their own expense. Products that are certified biological are usually more expensive, but their purity warrants the extra cost.

Many companies manufacture vapor-distilled essential oils, but the product available to you contains about 1 percent of that distillate, and the rest may be diluted with turpentine or alcohol.

Since essential oils are used in such minute doses, these diluents may not be harmful except to those with sensitivities or allergies to these substances. A label saying "100% guaranteed pure" does not ensure a pure product. All it is saying is that the extract itself—the essential oil—is pure, but it could be diluted.

Best choice: 100% guaranteed pure and botanically certified products ensure a consistent product. The chemical makeup of essential oils is difficult to pin down, since it depends on many environmental factors, but if a product offers the aforementioned guarantee, then it is properly distilled and undiluted. Generally, European essential oils are superior because they are subjected to strict regulatory standards established by government regulations.

Cold-Pressed Extraction to Yield Vegetable Oils

In cold-pressed extraction, oils are extracted from vegetables on an endless screw press—a press that squeezes the plant material between two metal plates. Usually the plant parts are first minced—though sometimes they are used whole—and then placed between the two metal plates of the endless screw press. These two plates close together like a jaw and squeeze the oil from the plant parts. This oil is collected in a vat installed under the press. Cold-pressed extraction occurs at temperatures not exceeding 85°F, or 32°C.

The advantage of cold-pressed extraction is that it occurs at low temperatures that will not destroy the nutrients contained in vegetables; food nutrients are particularly susceptible to damage from heat and light. In a sense, cold-pressed extraction yields a pure product because all it does is compress the vegetable.

Cold-pressed vegetable oils are far more nourishing than heat-extracted oils. But the consumer must be wary and read the fine print. Some manufacturers add chemical antioxidants, which prevent a product from deteriorating, or they bleach, blanch, deodorize, and discolor the product. These processes, known as re-fining procedures, destroy the active principles of the products. In addition, they may cause reactions within the substances that create noxious by-products. An oil that is labeled "extra virgin" is a cold-pressed oil that is completely unrefined, from organic sources, and certified biological.

Best choice: extra-virgin oil—choose the highest-quality cold-pressed oil commercially available. The flavor and texture of this oil reflects its pure quality.

Lyophilized Herb Capsules

High-quality herb capsules contain lyophilized herbs. These are herbs that have been freeze-dried and then subjected to a high-vacuum pressure immediately before they are encapsulated. This process ensures that the active components of the herbs are not destroyed and that their chemical structure remains intact. Lyophilized herbs are much more potent than simple dehy-drated herbs because the process is immediate and quick, pre-venting the alteration or destruction of active ingredients found in plants.

Many studies have indicated that the chemicals responsible for the therapeutic properties of plants were maintained when the plants were freeze-dried and lost when the plants were sim-ply air-dried. For example, two studies published in the presti-gious American Pharmaceutical Association's scientific edition of the *Journal of Pharmaceutical Science* in 1960 and 1961 com-pared the therapeutic activity of digitalis (*Digitalis purpurea;* leaves). It was found that the moisture present in leaves that had been air-dried at between 85°F and 100°F caused the break-down of glycosides—compounds that would have contributed therapeutic activity for cardiac conditions. Freezing the digitalis, however, prevented this breakdown, preserving and increasing the therapeutic activity of digitalis.

A similar pharmacological study showed that freeze-drying

dandelion root maintained high therapeutic potency by preserving the constituent compounds found in the living plant.

Best choice: organically produced dehydrated herbs that have been lyophilized. Such products are usually much more expensive than ordinary dehydrated herbs because the procedure is costly and requires sophisticated equipment.

Peptide-Bonded Amino Acids

When you hear the term "peptide-bonded," it is usually in relation to amino acids. A peptide bond links two amino acids by joining their nitrogen amide (NH_2) and carboxyl group ($COOH$). An amino acid is a small nitrogen-containing molecule; amino acids are the building blocks of proteins. There are 22 amino acids. Amino acids are arranged in chains, and peptide-bonded amino acids prepared in a laboratory are arranged in chains that contain 2 or 3 amino acids.

Amino acids are obtained when proteins break down during digestion. The human body can manufacture all but 8 of the 22 amino acids. These 8 amino acids are called essential amino acids and must be supplemented, like vitamins in the diet. Peptide-bonded amino acids usually come from protein substances that are digested by the pancreas or from plant or animal protein broken down by the pancreatic enzyme.

Proteins are absorbed by the body as complexes. Amino acid complexes are composed of two or three amino acids strung together. Studies have shown that peptide-bonded amino acids are more efficiently processed by the body than free-form amino acids. A free-form amino acid is a single amino acid, as opposed to the amino acid complex in the peptide-bonded amino acids. Both types of amino acids are available as tablets or in a powdered form that can be mixed into beverages. The difference lies in the way the body utilizes each type. Studies have shown that crystalline single amino acids draw water into the intestine, causing cramping, irritation, and diarrhea, and seriously interfering with the performance and absorption of the amino acid. More of the amino acid passes through the system, damaging it, than is absorbed and assimilated into muscle mass. Peptide-bonded amino acids ease protein synthesis, which enhances growth and muscle mass, performance, endurance, and recuperation.

Amino acids are generally taken by body builders or prescribed by physicians for specific conditions. In general, the body builder or health-conscious individual will take a combination of amino acids, whereas physicians may prescribe specific amino acids to treat deficiencies. These applications of amino acids are discussed in greater detail in chapter 9. Similarly, branched-chain amino acids (BCAA) are a direct source of energy and nourishment for muscles. A BCAA is an amino acid complex, a natural complex of leucine, isoleucine, and valine, the essential amino acids.

Best choice: peptide-bonded amino acids. These acids are better absorbed, more easily digested and subsequently assimilated more efficiently than free-form amino acids.

Chelated Minerals

In chelation, a mineral is bound to an amino acid. In the body, a single free-form mineral must bind to an amino acid. By consuming an already-bound mineral, the body saves energy and avoids unnecessary biochemical reactions that promote free radicals. A chelated mineral will be more easily assimilated right away because it is in a form that is ready to be processed by the body, rather than in a preliminary form that the body must modify before absorbing. Chelated minerals therefore are much more efficient than free-form minerals.

Best choice: chelated minerals. Chelated minerals act quickly, whereas free-form minerals are often lost in the body's biochemical processes. The breaking down and modifying of minerals often takes so long that the mineral passes right through the digestive tract without being absorbed.

Mineral Complexes

Mineral complexes are minerals that are joined to an acid; most of the time they are joined to a Krebs cycle acid. The Krebs cycle, otherwise referred to as cellular respiration, is a series of biochemical reactions that release energy, which enables the cell to do its work within the biosystem. The binding of a mineral to a Krebs cycle acid enhances the efficacy of a mineral by providing a vehicle for it. Uniting a mineral with an acid in a mineral complex ensures that the mineral will be properly metabolized. The mineral complex provides two bonuses: it helps the metabolism of proteins, carbohydrates, and fats, and it neutralizes lactic acid. Lactic acid causes muscle spasms, excessive sweating, and pain—all factors that suck energy from the body, decreasing endurance and contributing further pain and discomfort. These bonuses are especially important for athletes and all active people because the body is saving energy, which can be used for greater performance.

Best choice: mineral complexes, which are far more efficient than free-form minerals. In combination with chelated minerals, mineral complexes are unparalleled for efficacy and absorption in the body.

A Comparison of Tablets and Capsules

Even when the manufacturing process of a remedy or supplement is flawless, the final form of the product is also important, since it will affect its efficacy. For this reason, the major differences between tablets and capsules are worth discussing.

In the manufacturing of tablets, many additives, known as excipients, must be added. These are either:

—*Binders*—substances that help keep the ingredients in the tablet together.

—*Fillers*—substances that increase the size of the tablet when micro-quantities of active ingredients are used.

—*Solubility agents*—substances needed to help the tablet dissolve.

—*Lubricants*—substances that prevent the ingredients from sticking to the machine that produces the tablets.

—*Coatings*—substances that ease passage of pills during swallowing.

To make a tablet, tremendous pressure is needed, and this high level of pressure destroys many active ingredients. Often tablets are almost completely devoid of active ingredients. Studies have revealed some tablets to be insoluble in the digestive tract. X rays have shown a week's worth of tablets undissolved in the colon. Similar studies have shown that tablets can irritate the digestive tract, especially the stomach, and can cause constipation. Tablets are not a vehicle of choice for most active substances. Minerals, for instance, are stable compounds in the form of a supplement, but once inside the body, they become very reactive. In tablet form, minerals are often lost in the body, unable to reach their destination. If they do not reach their destination during the digestive process, they will not be assimilated and consequently the tablet will pass through the body slowly. This slow trek through the body not only neutralizes the minerals but also causes the excipients to linger in the body, increasing the risk that free-radical biochemical reactions will take place and that foreign substances will be left inside the body and will have to be eliminated.

Side effects such as constipation and indigestion associated with tablets have been clearly established, but some high-quality tablets do exist, and some products, such as sublingual products, must be taken in the form of a tablet. Most sublingual (under the tongue) tablets are pure and contain no excipients.

Capsules contain many fewer excipient substances. Certain low-grade capsules may contain fillers because companies that manufacture only one size of capsule must fill the rest of the capsule with substances like wheat or rice fillings. But coatings, binders, or pressure are not required to produce a capsule. Moreover, capsules are easier to swallow than tablets and are easier for the body to digest, because once swallowed, the capsule breaks apart, freeing its ingredients. The only excipient (unless the capsule contains low-grade ingredients or fillers) is the gelatin capsule itself. The body requires little energy to break down this tiny amount of gelatin. Some companies produce capsules tailored to the amount of active ingredient they contain, yielding an even smaller dose of gelatin. Capsules are convenient for those who have throat problems and need to take liquids, because they can be easily taken apart and their contents added to liquids. Since the source of gelatin of all capsules is animal, vegetarians can separate the capsule and add the ingredients to their food or beverages.

Foods and beverages can sometimes interfere with absorption of capsules, but this depends on the contents of the capsule, not on the gelatin capsule. For example, *a zinc supplement taken with an iron supplement will bind to the iron and carry it out of the body, reducing the intake of zinc and using up the iron as well as some of the body's energy.* The same reasoning advises against taking ginseng after eating vegetables and fruit and after drinking citrus drinks. The vitamin C in these foods depletes the ginseng and cancels its benefits. This interrelation between substances can be avoided by taking supplements at different times during the day, or by taking time-released products.

Time-released products are available as capsules or as tablets. They control the release of the active ingredients contained in the capsule or in the tablet. *Because the elements in a time-released product are liberated at different intervals after the ingestion of the capsule or tablet, interactions between antagonistic elements can be avoided.* This controlled-release mechanism is accomplished biochemically, causing the active ingredients to dissolve and to be released into the bloodstream at different intervals after ingestion. There are several methods of manufacturing time-released products, but these are beyond the scope of this book. Each method is specific to the product, and generally to the manufacturer of that product. There have not been any recorded cases of sensitivity to time-released products, but if you are concerned, you can contact the pharmaceutical division of the manufacturer for the biochemical specifications of its product.

Supplements are only now beginning to appear in capsule form, and only a handful of companies are putting vitamins and minerals in capsule form. Usually, these companies have a specific line of supplements in capsule form that comprises all the products in their line. In general, supplements in capsules are more expensive.

Best choice: capsules, because they are easier to swallow and contain fewer or no excipient substances.

To test the quality of your capsules, place one capsule in a 200°F oven. If the capsule turns a different color or shows a prism of colors, the capsule is not made of gelatin, but of plastic. Plastic capsules are rare, since the crackdown on health products; nevertheless, capsules from unfamiliar companies should be checked, because plastic is not good for you!

Liquid Health Products

Liquid products are beneficial because the active principles are in solution. Some active principles form precipitates—crystals—that can cause kidney ailments; such precipitates do not form in solution. Moreover, products that come in a liquid form are very potent because they require little digestion. Products that often come in liquid form are yeast tonics from plasmolyzed yeast, which are combined with orange juice and malt. Herbal extracts are liquid solutions containing 10 to 50 percent alcohol. Hydrolysates are liquids made up mostly of water, with a small percentage of plant extract. Some supplements, such as vitamins, can be found in liquid form. The old varieties suspended vitamins in malt, and some even contained alcohol. Today's new breed suspends its vitamins in liquid lecithin, vegetable glycerine, or purified water.

FOR FURTHER READING

Ali, S. E. F. "Study of the Lipid Fraction of Freeze-dried Dandelion Root." *Journal of Pharmaceutical Science* 51 (1962).

Goldblith and Karel, *Advances in Freeze-drying Lyophilisation*. Paris: Hernman, 1966.

Lohle, E.; Haussinger, D.; and Gerok, W. "Bioavailability of Zinc from Zinc-histidine Complexes. 1. Comparison with Zinc Sulfate in Healthy Men." *American Journal of Nutrition* (1987).

Lorenzi, G., and Cogoli, A. "Effect of Plasmolysed Yeast Preparations on Cellular Functions." *Swiss Biotech*, 3 (1985).

Schwarzenbach, Hans, Fritz. "Evaluation of 1140 Medical Practitioners' reports on the Efficacy of 11 Preparations in the Bio-Strath Range." *Swiss Pharma*, 1 (1979).

FOUR

Homeopathy

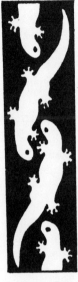

WHAT IS HOMEOPATHY?

In simple terms, homeopathy is the practice of curing like with like. A substance that duplicates the symptoms of a patient's illness is given in a diluted form, to provoke the body to heal itself. Homeopathic remedies do not add to symptoms, nor do they attack them; they act on the entire biosystem at the body's own pace, mostly at the bioenergetic level.

A homeopathic remedy is catalogued according to its "drug picture." This "drug picture" describes the effects of the remedy on a healthy person. These effects are matched to diseases that induce the same symptoms. For example, *Larrea mexicana*, a plant found in the arid regions of Northern Mexico, California, and Texas, has provoked, in clinical trials, reddening and itching of the skin, sneezing, and swelling of the eyes and face. It is used as a homeopathic remedy to treat hay fever and allergies because it reproduces the symptoms of these afflictions in a healthy person. The logic behind using like to cure like is that an infinitesimal dose of a substance that will induce symptoms of an illness in the body will cause the body to fight the illness, pushing the body towards normal metabolism and health.

Within the medical community, homeopathy is considered a natural healing method, but it follows an allopathic principle. Small amounts of toxins are used to reverse the course of a disease, in the same way the allopathic process of immunization works. For example, vaccinations increase the body's resistance to foreign cells by providing the antigen that will destroy them. In simple terms, the process of immunization involves the introduction of antigens that lock onto the walls of foreign cells, penetrate, and neutralize the virus. Vaccines introduce the antigens, which must be specific in order to fit foreign cells.

Orthodox allopathic medicine discovered that very few antigens are needed to neutralize a virus in the body. As few as 23 antigens may be required to neutralize 600 viral cells. Homeopathy pushes the body into healing itself in the same way. The difference is that homeopathic remedies are taken from natural biosystems that contribute an energy pattern that is compatible with that of the cells, whereas vaccines are made from killed viruses.

THE ORIGINS OF HOMEOPATHY

The birth and evolution of modern homeopathy is attributed to German physician Samuel Hahnemann. Hahnemann was a professor at Leipzig University in the eighteenth century. Hahnemann disagreed with many of the allopathic medical approaches of his day and could not accept the lack of suitable cures for many ailments. With the help of some of his students, Hahnemann tested several remedies, mostly from plant sources, and began to catalogue the reactions to these remedies. He classified his results according to the principle of like cures like, and expanding upon it, established the law of similars.

In his classification, Hahnemann paid as much attention to the emotional and mental symptoms as he did to the physical. He then began to treat patients, giving them remedies that would reproduce their illness. The results bore out his law of similars. The patients experienced an initial worsening of the illness, called the healing crisis, followed by a complete cure. In his writings, Hahnemann concluded that by applying his law of similars and prescribing substances that artificially reproduced the illness in the individual, he was stimulating the body's natural defenses.

THE PREPARATION OF HOMEOPATHIC REMEDIES

Homeopathic remedies are dilutions of plant extracts. Sometimes other organic substances from animal or mineral sources, such as snake venom, sulfur, or calcium, are used. The original extract is a tincture. As described in chapter 1, a plant tincture is prepared by macerating a plant in alcohol. This initial tincture, called the mother tincture, is designated by the symbol Ø. Solid matter such as a mineral is pulverized and diluted with lactose to form a tablet. The mother tincture is diluted several times to prepare the actual homeopathic remedy to be administered. If you have a lactose intolerance, you should take liquid homeopathic remedies, as all homeopathic tablets are made with lactose.

The process of dilution is the most important part of preparing homeopathic remedies. One drop of the mother tincture is placed in either 9 or 99 parts of water and mechanically shaken, or succussed. This violent shaking of the solution is done in the laboratory by a succussion device. Manual shaking of the solution is not enough to disperse the atoms. When the solution is diluted with 9 parts water, the remedy is labeled with a numerical value, signaling the extent of the dilution, followed by an *X*. If the dilution is made with 100 parts of water, the numerical value will be followed by a *C*. For example, a milliliter of mother tincture diluted once using 9 parts water will be labeled 1X. A mother tincture diluted once with 99 parts water will be labeled 1C. The solution must be succussed after each dilution.

The solid or mineral pulverizations are diluted in the same

proportions as the liquid tincture, except that lactose is used instead of water, and tablets result as the homeopathic remedy rather than liquids. Liquid-water dilutions are used directly as homeopathic remedies, or they can be used to coat milk-sugar capsules, which the patient then takes according to a physician's instructions.

The process of diluting homeopathic remedies is called potentization. *Unlike allopathic drugs, homeopathic remedies become more potent the more they are diluted.* To understand this process, it is important to understand how chemical quantities are measured. The quantity of a chemical substance is measured in moles. A mole is essentially the mass of a substance that is numerically equal to the mass of the molecules it contains. Molecules are composed of atoms. In chemical proportions, the concentration of a substance is measured against Avogadro's number. Avogadro was an Italian physicist who set the number of molecules in a mole at 6.023×10^{23}. Homeopathic remedies are so diluted that they often do not contain even one atom of the original substance. Suppose you are diluting a substance with 99 parts of water. As in the sample above, after 12 dilutions with 99 parts of water, you will have a solution with a concentration of 10^{-24}. This is under Avogadro's number $(10^{23})^{x-24}$, leaves 0.1, telling you that the dilution does not contain one atom of the mother tincture. Yet homeopaths show time and again that the higher a remedy's dilution, the more potent its effect in the body.

Homeopathic remedies are at the opposite end of the numerical scale from allopathic drugs. Allopathic drugs must be administered in concentrations that are great enough to saturate the bloodstream. In contrast, homeopathic remedies rarely contain even one molecule of the original herbal extract. This is the main reason homeopathic drugs are not readily accepted as a medical treatment. In fact, they are often considered by allopathic physicians to act as a palliative for psychosomatic illnesses. However, the curative properties of homeopathic remedies are due to their energy patterns.

THE ENERGY PATTERN OF A HOMEOPATHIC REMEDY

All biosystems have energy patterns. An energy pattern causes the system to vibrate at its optimal level. When there are disturbances in the energy pattern, the biosystem will suffer damage, initially at the cellular level (because cells receive information from their surroundings), then at the levels of organs and systems. When there is not even an atom of the original tincture left in the dilution of a homeopathic remedy and still practitioners get results, the only thing left must be the energy imprint of the original substance. Recent research with nuclear magnetic resonance techniques have shown these drugs to contain the energy impact of the original substance.

Just as studies with the AMI machine and the Voll machine have confirmed the existence of a cardinal energy flowing through the human body, experiments with holographic equipment have demonstrated that plants and other biological substances have their own energy imprint.

A holographic picture is a three-dimensional representation of an object. In simple terms, a hologram is a pattern caused by the convergence of two light beams that is captured on photographic film. Biologically, cloning an organism by taking cells from one part of a biosystem would seem to work on a holographic principle. Evidence in support of this theory was presented in 1940 by neuroanatomist Harold Burr, who set out to measure the bioenergy fields in a biosystem. His first experiments involved the shape of electrical fields surrounding salamanders, and the bioenergetic growth fields of salamanders. Analyzing the microvoltage levels, Burr found that *the hologram of a salamander, regardless of which stage of development the salamander was in when the holograph was taken, was shaped like an adult animal.* Burr also discovered that the electrical field contained an electrical axis that was aligned with the brain and the spinal cord. His studies eventually led him to find that this electrical axis originated in the unfertilized egg. Burr carried out similar experiments measuring the bioenergy fields of seedlings and leaves. Using the same holographic principles, he measured the electrical field around a sprout and found it to be the shape of the adult plant. This confirmed the observations Burr had found with salamanders, suggesting that a predetermined growth template was generated by an organism's electromagnetic field.

Similar results were found in the experiments of Russian scientist Semyon Kirlian. Kirlian used holographic equipment to measure the electrical fields of the human body. His results were manifested visually by a discharge of sparks which are known as the Kirlian aura. Both these scientists found, after further exploration, that diseases produce significant changes in the electromagnetic fields of the body.

These experiments revealed that there is exciting diagnostic potential in electrographic recording techniques. The AMI machine and the Voll machine are two devices that make use of these techniques. The Voll machine possesses a holder that allows homeopathic remedies to be inserted, making it easy to match the remedy to the altered electrical field of the body. A more sophisticated, meridian-based diagnostic device that is gaining recognition is the Interro. The Interro is a computer that contains the energy pattern imprints of hundreds of homeopathic remedies stored in a memory bank. Whereas the Voll machine needs the homeopathic remedies to be introduced physically, the Interro automatically matches a homeopathic remedy with the patient's energy balance.

These devices, mainly used by homeopaths and naturopaths, give us further evidence that homeopathic remedies possess the energy pattern imprint of their original substances in the mother tincture. They appear to work at the bioenergetic level to realign the patient's altered energy pattern, rather than to intervene at the cellular level. As a result, homeopathic remedies do not interfere with body processes and thus do not induce entropy. Instead, they allow the biosystem to find its biochemical balance at the body's pace, without inducing side effects. This is a basic principle of natural healing.

Another experiment giving credence to the matching of frequencies between remedy and illness concerns the healing of fractured bones. A study published in *Medical World News* in 1978 revealed that a fractured bone is influenced by its electromagnetic fields. Changes in frequencies surrounding the injured bone influence the "behavior" of the bone and whether its cells will produce new calcium or bone tissue will break down.

Because homeopathic remedies work at the bioenergetic level of the biosystem, they can influence altered energy patterns caused by mental and emotional upsets. Minor illnesses often are expressions of more serious conditions brewing within the biosystem and are due to the altered energy patterns caused by mental, emotional, environmental, and even spiritual factors. By acting on the energy pattern, homeopathic remedies can realign the cardinal energy of the biosystem, cure the system of its "warning illness," and prevent further illnesses. Since only the proper frequency will move an electron to an orbit of higher frequency (as described in chapter 1), introducing the proper frequency with a homeopathic remedy provokes the body to oscillate at its healthy frequency and to heal itself.

Part of the healing process involves the discharge of toxins. Sometimes homeopathic remedies cause an initial worsening of the illness, called the "healing crisis." The severity of this crisis generally corresponds to the dilution of the remedy. Usually this exacerbation of symptoms occurs because the body is eliminating toxins. We could go so far as to say that the temporary exacerbation of symptoms is a proof that healing is occurring in the body.

Since the homeopathic remedy is pure energy, it realigns the energy pattern of the body. This readjustment is like an explosion that pushes the body toward a state of health. During the healing crisis, there may be extreme fatigue and general malaise for a few days.

Like other natural healing techniques, homeopathy does not simply relieve symptoms but aims to cure illness. Since homeopathic remedies act at the bioenergetic level, they are effective with such chronic or recurring illness as arthritic conditions, allergies, and ear infections, and for the physical manifestations of emotional states. Allergies like hayfever, for example, are an expression of an overzealous immune system, which overreacts to foreign substances. Similarly, a condition like arthritis means the immune system is overreacting to one's own body cells. In contrast, when the immune system is in a languid state and not carrying out its duty of attacking foreign cells, infections occur. Homeopathic remedies, though, work on the immune system itself by realigning the body's energy patterns. In this way, the body's biological balance is restored without accosting other systems not previously affected by the illness, as allopathic drugs do.

Homeopathic remedies act to connect the body's healing energies with its illness. When such conditions as pollution, stress, preservatives, and toxins in foods cause an illness that proceeds almost like a separate entity from the body, homeopathic remedies realign the body with the illness, allowing the biosystem to start a chain reaction of biochemical processes towards recovery.

THE EMOTIONAL LINK

Homeopathic doctors emphasize the emotional connection that homeopathic remedies seem to possess. Although this connection has not been proven, it is possible that emotions have a particular frequency. We have all experienced fluttering feelings in the stomach when we are nervous or scared. It has been established that this physiological response to an emotional state is caused by the production of epinephrine—a hormone secreted into the bloodstream by the medullas of the adrenal glands. Here, once again, is evidence of the relationship between the surroundings and action of cells and the subsequent state of the entire biosystem. In order for the cells of the medullas to release epinephrine (also called adrenalin), they must receive a signal from the brain. These signals are electrical impulses that arrive via the sympathetic nervous system. The signal causes electrochemical changes in the biosystem, which then manifest themselves as physical conditions. For example, the release of adrenalin when you are scared causes your heart to race. It is the chemicals released by the body that cause the physical symptoms, but the initial reaction, the one that caused the release of the chemical (in this case called a transmitter) is set off by an electrical impulse—a frequency. Homeopathic remedies may cause such sparks to set off electrochemical reactions, and in this sense, they may be said to treat at the emotional level.

When Hahnemann collected substances for homeopathic remedies, he considered the emotional and mental nature of the illness, which he incorporated into the symptom complex of the remedy. He believed that a physical condition would affect the mental and emotional character of a patient, and in some instances, the emotional and mental condition of a patient manifested physical ailments. British physician and bacteriologist Edward Bach elaborated on Hahnneman's theory linking disease and emotion. During his work as a bacteriologist, Bach investigated the types of bacteria found in the gastrointestinal tract of persons suffering from chronic ailments. The association of certain types of bacteria with certain ailments was so distinct that Bach decided to immunize patients against the type of bacteria present. He reasoned that inoculating his patients with vaccines made from a specific type of bacteria should move the body to eject the associated microorganisms.

Bach diluted the bacteria found in the intestines of his patients beyond Avogadro's number, so as not to inject physical pathogens into his patients. These dilutions of pathogens are called bionosodes. Bionosodes are essentially homeopathic dilutions made from diseased tissue. Bach's vaccines were effective in relieving his patients' infections. However, irritation and inflammation frequently occurred at the site of injection, which proved to be uncomfortable for the patient. Bach remedied this phenomenon by diluting the bacteria, formulating a homeo-pathic remedy that patients could take sublingually. These homeopathic preparations were very successful in relieving chronic ailments.

Altogether, Bach had prepared seven dilutions, from the seven different bacteria he had discovered in patients with dif-ferent diseases. During Bach's treatment of his patients with these seven bionosodes, he discovered that a distinct personality type was linked to each bacterium. In fact, he considered that he was dealing with seven distinct personalities, not seven different illnesses. Each personality type reacted to a disease, any disease, the same way, with the same state of mind and outlook. Bach concluded that *specific personality types predisposed patients to spe-cific illnesses.* From this conclusion, he proceeded to link bionosodes to a patient's mental and emotional characteristics.

Part of Hahnemann's cataloguing of homeopathic remedies included the emotional and mental effects of a particular rem-edy. This emotional link of homeopathic remedies with the biosystem is what makes them valuable in treating chronic dis-eases and the stress-induced ailments so common today.

HOW TO RECOGNIZE A HOMEOPATHIC REMEDY

Homeopathic remedies are dilutions. Packaging reveals the de-gree of the dilution as an X or a C, as explained at the beginning of this chapter. Herbal remedies that claim to be homeopathic but do not identify the degree of their dilution are clearly not ho-meopathic; they are diluted herbal extracts that do not have the same action in the body. Herbal remedies indicate the concen-tration of plant tincture in percentages—for example, 0.05 per-cent of a particular tincture—or carry the symbol $\emptyset$ indicating that it is the mother tincture, meaning that an undiluted tincture of the whole plant is used in the herbal remedy.

Although herbal formulae and homeopathic preparations may at times look the same, it is important to realize their therapeutic differences and to recognize the difference in their formulation, because each of these remedy types works on a very different premise. Herbal remedies target physiological avenues. Their formulations are based on the therapeutic properties of plants and on whether they are decongestant, sedative, anti-inflammatory, and so on. *Homeopathic remedies are based on the symptom portrait, and they do not contribute therapeutic properties to the individual but rather reproduce the symptoms of a disease to provoke the body into a healing state.* A true homeopathic remedy acts at the "vibrational" level and contains no illness-causing components.

ABSORPTION OF HOMEOPATHIC REMEDIES

Homeopathic remedies are absorbed through the mucous membranes, where they can reach the bloodstream. It is for this reason that instructions require some tablets to be dissolved under the tongue. Likewise, liquid remedies should remain in the mouth for about one minute before they are swallowed. As homeopathic remedies are often altered or destroyed by gastric secretion, they should be taken fifteen minutes to half an hour before meals. Homeopathic remedies should be taken only upon the recommendation of a homeopathic physician, and doses should be strictly followed. Because homeopathic remedies work at the energy level, proper treatment with these remedies is a most important factor in therapy. *Dosing homeopathic remedies requires many years of experience and should not be attempted by a layperson.* Disrupted bioenergetic patterns can lead to serious physical illnesses. Properly prescribed, homeopathic remedies redirect bioenergetic patterns. Indiscriminate use of these products is very risky.

Like all natural remedies, homeopathic remedies should not be consumed with other types of remedies, especially allopathic drugs. Homeopathic remedies help provoke the body to realign its energy pattern to a healthy state. Other drugs may counteract the effect of the homeopathic remedy.

DANGERS ASSOCIATED WITH HOMEOPATHIC REMEDIES

Because homeopathic remedies cause specific disease symptoms within the body, it is essential that you know exactly what your symptoms are, the symptom portrait of the homeopathic remedy, and what it has been classified to treat. Symptomology is a precise science. Also, similar symptoms can indicate very different conditions. For these reasons, it is important to leave homeopathic treatment to the homeopathic physician. One symptom left out of series can mean the difference between illness and wellness! In addition, the energy pattern of the homeopathic remedy must be compatible with that of the patient, and thus different homeopathic strengths must be matched with different patients. This precision matching requires years of experience and is another reason why homeopathy should be left up to the professional physician. Not only must the remedy match the symptoms exactly, it must be prescribed in the right dilution to do its work effectively.

FOR FURTHER READING

Burr, H. S. *The Fields of Life.* New York: Ballantine Books, 1972.
Gerber, Richard. *Vibrational Medicine.* New Mexico: Bear & Co., 1988.
"Healing Intransigent Fractures." *Medical World News (April 17, 1978).*
Kirlian, S., and Kirlian, V. "Photography and Visual Observations by Means of High Frequency Currents." *Journal of Scientific and Applied Photography* 6 (1961).
Mallikarjun, S. "Kirlian Photography in Cancer Diagnosis." *Osteopathic Physician* 6 (1961).

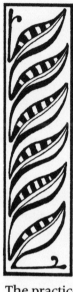

FIVE

Naturopathy

WHAT IS NATUROPATHY?

The practice of naturopathy is limited to the use of natural remedies and methods in the treatment of disease. Here "natural" refers strictly to nonsynthetic methods. This means no drugs and
no processed foods, and the most traditional naturopaths will
only subscribe to organic herbal formulas and foods. *Generally,
naturopathy will deal with an ailment by changing the diet, rather
than by administering a remedy.* Such processes as massage, hy-
drotherapy (massage with water jets), osteopathy (manipulation of the skeletal system), and other forms of physical manipulation are used instead of the molecular manipulation stimu-
lated by remedies. Macrobiotics is an important part of naturopathy. Macrobiotics incorporates much of the doctrine that food
is divided into yin and yang (female and male) and that foods
influence the physiological functioning and structure of the
body. A macrobiotic diet is a vegetarian diet that is thought to
hold the individual in balance with the cosmos.

Naturopathy uses any method that naturally catalyzes the

body processes. For instance, it will use massage to stimulate the circulation. There is never any type of infusion with chemicals. (In fact, those who strictly adhere to naturopathy will not even have freezing during dental procedures.) Sometimes essential oils are used in massage oils, and although we know that these penetrate the epithelium and infiltrate the bloodstream, they are accepted as natural remedies.

Traditional naturopathy follows the order of the universe. It is believed, as in Chinese medicine, that any part of the environment taken into the body will shape the internal environment of the body. The application of naturopathy balances the internal body with the external environment. This balance creates certain physical and mental states. By the same token, outgoing and incoming energies must be balanced. If the outgoing energy exceeds the incoming energy, certain organs may become overactive, resulting in chronic conditions. If outgoing energy becomes less than incoming energy, organs may become underactive, resulting in degenerative diseases.

Naturopathy believes that individuals have a predisposition to certain conditions as a result of factors received from their parents' reproductive cells. The physical manifestations of these factors are known as constitutions, whereas those created by our daily consumption of food and drink make up our condition. Naturopathy studies the interaction between one's constitution and condition, evaluating the antagonistic and complemental relationships between the physical and the mental aspects of each during diagnosis. In naturopathy it is believed that manifestation of illness occurs because of the change in relationship between the opposing factors and tendencies. Illness can be counteracted through a change in lifestyle and diet, for these are what form the antagonistic and complemental relationships that shape the internal environment of the biosystem. These changes can be as simple as a change in attitude, possibly afforded by a therapy such as rebirth. Rebirth is a technique that teaches a person renewal of the spirit, mind, and body. It is an extension of a 17th-century theory based on the cyclical regeneration of the universe and its beings.

Naturopathic methods are very time-consuming and do not always apply readily to a normal working lifestyle. Hours a day may be devoted to walks, meditation, and cooking of a special macrobiotic diet, which involves lengthy preparation of fresh organic vegetables.

NATUROPATHIC REMEDIES

Naturopathy is based on the belief that each substance and each effect has its opposite in nature. Poisonous substances have their antidotes, and a geographic region possesses curative substances for its illness somewhere in its wild countryside.

In the early 18th century, the Reverend Stone had great faith in this belief. He postulated that an antidote to rheumatism, which a great many of his parishioners suffered from, existed in nature within the immediate vicinity. In 1763 his faith lead him to discover willow bark, which may not have cured rheumatism but did alleviate rheumatic pain. This event heralded major changes in medicine. The controversy between holistic approaches, which were the methods of medicine of the past, and the invention of laboratory derivatives of natural substances, came to a head, and within a few decades, chemists had formulated acetyl salicylic acid, commonly known as aspirin, from willow bark.

The germ theory further pushed the old holistic ways out of medicine and ushered in what we now call allopathic medicine and drugs. The focus on healing the whole individual was replaced by the theory that each disease had a well-defined cause and could be controlled or cured by attacking the causative agent. This in turn led to treatment of only the affected parts of the body. Naturopathic practitioners shuddered at the thought of the consequences of attacking the causative agent. They claimed that this mode of treatment was more likely to worsen patients' condition than to cure them.

Naturopathy treats the individual as a whole biosystem attached to a total environment. All factors, both internal and external, are considered in diagnosis and treatment. Although some allopathic diagnostic tests (like blood tests) are used by naturopaths, emphasis is placed on avoiding stress. If the test will stress the individual, exacerbating his or her symptoms, it will probably not be done. Furthermore, only natural substances that do not leave residues, such as organically produced herbal extracts, are used in treatment. Instead of prescribing vitamins, a naturopath will formulate an organic or macrobiotic diet. Complete and tailored regimes are prepared in naturopathic treatment, including diet, exercise, stress management, lifestyle changes, and so on. In fact, naturopathy is a really holistic treatment, with greatest emphasis on natural living.

Naturopathy and other systems of natural healing are often less cut and dried than allopathic medicine; their approach to conditions is broad and cannot efficiently be governed by any kind of licensing board. Because many disciplines enter into natural healing, such as nutrition, biochemistry, osteopathy, and counseling, it is difficult to establish professional standards to be strictly followed by natural practitioners. However, associations of each discipline, such as holistic medicine, nutrition, and osteopathy, provide some form of convergence for natural healing practitioners. They allow for standards of training and for the exchange of information and networking to bring the most recent and best-documented forms of treatments to the public.

Phytotherapy, the treatment of illness using plants, is a big part of naturopathy. Herbs are also used as sources of vitamins and minerals, rather than the prepared or synthetic versions. *In naturopathy, the herbalist replaces the pharmacist and prepares herbal combinations for specific problems and individuals, rather than prescribing a general formula you might buy at the health food store.*

Bone manipulation, such as osteopathy, and massage therapy, such as orthotherapy, are also major forms of naturopathic treatment. These treatments tend to realign or activate specific areas of the body and are usually used in conjunction with herbs (single herbs, tinctures, or extracts) as an adjunct to the primary treatment. For example, a back problem might be treated with either osteopathy or orthotherapy, depending on the nature of the problem, and supported by herbs that improve the immune system, such as echinacae, and perhaps nettle to increase the mineral profile of the blood and dandelion to remove acids from the blood. In this case, the sore back would be seen as being aggravated by stress. Thus the passage therapy would be used to correct the musculoskeletal problem, and the herb therapy would be used to reinforce the body's defense system.

FOR FURTHER READING

Dubos, René. *Mirage of Health: Utopias, Progress, and Biological Change.* New Brunswick and London: Rutgers University Press, 1987.

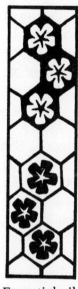

SIX

Health Uses
of Essential Oils

ESSENTIAL OILS IN HISTORY

Essential oils are sometimes referred to as aromatic compounds, and the use of essential oils in therapy is called aromatherapy. Aromatherapy involves the administration of essential oils by three routes: topically to the skin; internally, by ingestion; and externally, by inhalation therapy.

Aromatherapy dates back to antiquity, when essential oils were used as remedies by the Greeks and the Egyptians. They also used essential oils to produce fine perfumes, and it is this application of essential oils that has lasted throughout history. The ancient practice of aromatherapy was all but forgotten until its rebirth during the 16th and 17th centuries, when aromatherapy techniques were passed on to apprentices.

Modern-day aromatherapy is still practiced in Europe, where the manufacture of essential oils is big business as a result of the perfume industry. In Europe, aromatherapy is taught in much the same way as in ancient times; the information is passed along as a sort of apprenticeship. Often closed societies devoted to the production and study of applications of essential oils are formed, somewhat like the wineries of religious orders. From these societies have evolved many treatments using essential oils—from the treatment of emotional disorders to the use of essential oils in vibrational medicine. Today these ancient applications of aromatherapy are practiced and taught mostly in Europe by those closed societies, making it difficult to find people who are experienced with these substances. But most North American naturopathic physicians can refer you to such a person.

Today aromatherapy has gained ground in America. The success of the ancient therapy is starting to receive scientific verification as a result of recent experiments with essential oils. In 1980, Clegg and colleagues published an article in *Biochemical Pharmacology,* revealing that a chemical compound found in essential oil of orange could lower cholesterol. A terpene called limonene accomplished this by blocking the enzyme responsible for the laying down of cholesterol, which is how cholesterol-lowering drugs works. A 1987 study published in the *Journal of Toxicological and Environmental Health* showed that the terpene d-limonene activated the immune system in the defense against cancer. These studies have brought essential oils into the medical community. There is still much ground to cover, but the ancient treatments are being justified, and aromatherapy is sure to gain popularity in the next few years. Now researchers and experienced aromatherapists are teaching other medical professionals and continuing to investigate essential oils scientifically.

Of course, this newfound interest in essential oils means that there will be an influx of products on the market. Essential oils are both very specific and very complex substances that must be understood. They can also be dangerous, and products that are mere laboratory reproductions do not mimic the properties of the natural substances. Furthermore, commercial essential oils, both synthetically and naturally produced, may have been diluted with such questionable products as alcohol or turpentine. However, since essential oils are used in such minute doses, these diluents may not be harmful, except to individuals who have sensitivities and allergies to these products. For example, a person allergic to petrochemicals could become quite ill if using an essential oil diluted with turpentine. *Avoiding bargain prices is one of the best ways to avoid diluted products.*

WHAT IS AN ESSENTIAL OIL?

An essential oil is a fragrant liquid extracted from a plant through vapor distillation. This process is discussed in detail in chapter 3. Despite its name, an essential oil may or may not be of an oily consistency. An essential oil is part of the plant's immune system. During drought or other climatic changes, or if there are deficiencies in the soil, the plant's essential oil takes over to help the plant survive. In a sense, the essential oil acts as a sort of back-up system. The plant's increased production of essential oil under difficult conditions is demonstrated by the stronger fragrance of dried herbs than that of fresh plants. As the plant dries, it produces essential oil to compensate for the loss of water. *Analysis confirms that the amount of essential oil contained in a plant is inversely proportional to the amount of water in the plant.* We can also smell the difference between the cultured flower and the same variety grown in the wild. The wild variety has a stronger, more distinct odor than the cultured variety.

Today chemistry recognizes organic compounds as those that contain the element carbon. Even though chemists can make these organic carbon compounds in the laboratory, the historic division between inorganic and organic compounds has been retained. For convenience, this book refers to chemicals taken from living sources as organic and those manufactured in the laboratory as synthetic.

In discussing natural remedies, the difference between an organic compound and a synthetic compound lies in the substance's bioenergy. Since organic substances come from living sources that have an innate electromagnetic field that is distributed throughout the organism, the molecules obtained from that living system will hold this bioenergy. A synthetic compound will not have the bioenergy found in the organic substance, even if it is a perfect chemical replica of the organic compound.

The fact that essential oils come from nature does not make them harmless or less potent than manufactured chemicals. In fact, they are more potent than their synthetically produced counterparts because:

–They are more concentrated.

–They have an energy pattern that is more compatible with the energy pattern of the human body's cells.

The plant generates its essential oil through photosynthesis, a biochemical process that uses the sun's energy to split a water molecule into its component parts: oxygen and hydrogen. The sun's energy is transferred to the essential oil, making it a very active substance. A law of physics states that energy cannot be created or destroyed but only transformed, and the energy from the sun is transformed into biomagnetic energy within the essential oil.

The chemical composition of the essential oil depends on biochemical reactions called oxidation-reduction reactions, in which an electron from one molecule is passed to another molecule. When it starts out, the electron carries much energy, but as it is transferred, it loses energy to energy-rich compounds, which it helps form. In a plant these compounds carry energy to multicarbon compounds. These multicarbon compounds or carbon chains are the organic chemicals that make up essential oils. The energy used to create multicarbon chains in essential oils originates from the sun.

In some plant varieties, the multicarbon compounds settle in different parts of the plant. In these varieties, the chemical makeup of the essential oil will depend on which part of the plant is distilled. An essential oil is generally composed of three to five different groups of multicarbon compounds.

The chemical makeup of an essential oil depends on many

factors and changes with the life stage of the plant, the geographical location of the plant, the climactic conditions of the plant's environment, and the part of the plant used for the distillation (flowers, stems, roots, leaves, or bark).

LIFE STAGE OF THE PLANT

The chemical makeup of an essential oil changes with the life stage of the plant. You can see this change in the flowers of *Verbena officinalis*, whose magnificent perfume fills the air when they are in bloom, and whose terribly bitter odor is dispersed after the blooming period. This change occurs because the chemical makeup of verbena's essential oil changes with the plant's life stage as a result of biochemical reactions similar to our own hormone changes.

GEOGRAPHICAL LOCATION OF THE PLANT

Geographical location seems to cause the most striking change in an essential oil. Often this change is not detectable to the untrained nose. Chromatographic analysis taken from samples of essential oils distilled from plants of the same species, at exactly the same stage, but grown in different locations, have revealed different chemical compositions. They show multicarbon compounds in essential oils belonging to different chemical groups (ketone, ester, aldehyde, oxide, or terpene), which give specific properties to the essential oil.

Essential oil of rosemary is a good example of the different chemicals produced in the same species grown in different locations. The Latin name for true rosemary is *Rosmarinus officinalis*. The original wild variety that grows in the different parts of Europe contains an ester as its main chemical group and a ketone in almost equal proportions, whereas the same variety cultivated in a hothouse contains an oxide as its main chemical group. The same variety grown near the Mediterranean has a ketone as its main group and smells much more like camphor than the other essential oils of rosemary. *The differences in chemical composition of rosemary's essential oil when grown in different regions are shown below.*

FIG. EO-1 *Chemical compositions of three essential oils distilled from the same plant species, grown in different geographical locations.*

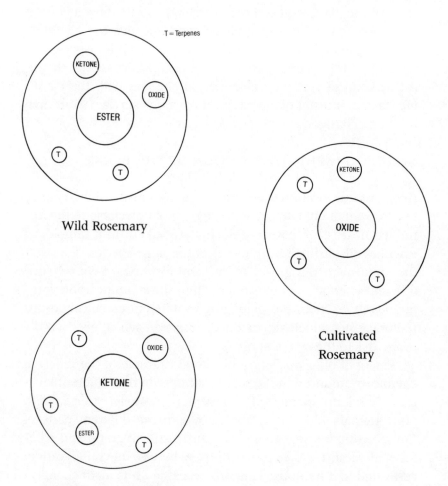

Wild Rosemary

Cultivated Rosemary

Mediterranean Rosemary

Wild varieties of some plants are sometimes successfully cultivated in hothouses without any alteration in their chemical makeup. The essential oils distilled from these plants possess the same chemical makeup contained in the transplanted original wild plant. But the properties of the essential oil from the cultivated plant will be weaker than those of the plant harvested from the wild. Essential oils distilled from wild plants that have been transplanted in hothouses are graded as "biological" or "organic" cultures. If the word "biological," or its abbreviation "bio," or the word "organic," or its abbreviation "org," appears on a label, then the essential oil is from a cultivated plant grown in a hothouse. Reputable companies will also include the geographic origin of the plant harvested from the wild and now cultured in a hothouse. For example, a label for essential oil of lavender might read: "Lavender, Provence. Org." This indicates this oil was distilled from true lavender *(Lavandula vera)*, originating from Provence in France, but cultivated in a hothouse. Although this type of information on a label is rare, it is necessary to know the chemical specificity of an essential oil. There are no regulations requiring that this information be placed on labels, but aromatherapists and those specialists studying, producing, and working with essential oils are lobbying to make this label information a prerequisite for commercial distribution.

CLIMACTIC CONDITIONS OF THE PLANT'S ENVIRONMENT

Changes in climate also cause chemical changes in the essential oils. Since the oil is an active part of the plant, it is affected by changes in soil chemistry caused by climate, by sun intensity and duration, by chemical changes of the ambient air due to pollution and climate, by temperature changes, and by rainfall. Thus, different chemical groups become more or less prominent under different climatic conditions.

Rarely is there only one chemical in an essential oil, and there are usually about ten chemical groups associated with essential oils. *Most essential oils contain a combination of between three and five main chemical groups, each of which has specific therapeutic properties.*

THE PLANT PART USED FOR EXTRACTION

Some essential oils are found within the entire plant, and therefore distilling them involves using the entire plant. For other oils, specific parts of the plant must be used in distillation. In some varieties, canal-like secreting organs contain the essential oils. These organs may be located in different parts of the plant, such as in the needlelike leaves of rosemary or in the flowers of lavender.

The multicarbon compounds produced from the oxidation-reduction reactions settle in different parts of the plant. For example, mint produces esters, which are found in the stem, and alcohols, which are found in the leaves. *The cedar tree produces two different essential oils. One produced from distillation of the leaves yields a dangerous substance that contains a poison, called thujone.* This essential oil is not "oily" and does not carry the characteristic odor of cedar wood. Essential oil of cedar bark is an oilier substance, with the traditional fragrance of cedar wood.

THE ESSENTIAL OILS' MAIN CHEMICAL GROUPS AND THEIR PROPERTIES

Aldehydes

These substances are anti-inflammatory, reducing swelling, especially of the skin. They are hypothermic, cooling by constricting blood vessels, and lowering arterial pressure. Applied topically (to the skin), they are astringent, causing the pores to contract. They are also bactericidal, killing bacteria.

Terpenes

These substances are bactericidal, fungicidal (killing fungus growths), and viricidal (killing viruses), and they strengthen the immune system. They can be a general tonic for the body.

Dienes

These substances are usually found in small proportions in essential oils. They are anticoagulant, preventing clotting of blood, and antispasmodic, preventing constriction of muscles. *Dienes are extremely active substances; therefore, essential oils that possess this chemical group are very effective.*

Alcohols

The properties of these substances depend on which chemical groups they are combined with. In general, an alcohol is astringent and may be a general tonic for the body.

Ethers

The compounds in this group are sedative, helping relax the entire body and inducing sleep. They are antispasmodic, as well as antidepressant, enhancing mood.

Oxides

These substances are mucinolytic, thinning mucous secretions—especially in the lungs and breathing passages. They are also decongestant, helping to dilate breathing passages to enhance air flow. They decongest arteries and veins, increasing the flow of blood.

Acids

The substances in this group are anti-inflammatory. They are also hypothermic, lowering body temperature by constricting blood vessels.

Esters

The substances in this group are antispasmodic, sedative, and tonic (physically or mentally invigorating), and they can stabilize the nervous system.

Phenols

The substances in this group are anthelmintic, expelling internal parasites. They are bactericidal, fungicidal, and germicidal, destroying bacteria, viruses, or protozoa (a phylum of small, single-celled or colonial organisms). *Phenols are highly toxic, and minute doses can produce reactions*. Phenols' properties are reversed at high doses. They are also hyperthermic, elevating body temperature by dilating blood vessels. This effect may also cause high blood pressure.

Ketones

The substances in this group are anticoagulant, sedative, and mucinolytic. Ketones are dangerous substances, because they are neurotoxic, corrupting the nervous system by poisoning and destroying nerves.

Clearly, some of these chemical groups are dangerous poisons, and indeed, *some essential oils are unsafe*. Essential oils must be knowledgeably administered in minute doses, usually two to seven drops per dose. Even poisons can be beneficial in minute doses. An example is essential oil of clove. It contains a great deal of the phenol eugenol, which causes uterine dilation and which may lead to abortion in pregnant women and animals. Some hospitals in France use essential oil of phenol to induce labor. As well, an appropriate dose of this essential oil can be useful in arresting certain bacterial and viral infections.

Since an essential oil may contain several compounds (usually between three and five), belonging to the above chemical groups, it is not possible to name its therapeutic properties by simply listing the properties associated with each group. Usually, a compound from one of the listed groups is present in a larger quantity than the others. The compound present in the greater quantity determines the "main group," and the essential oil is categorized and often named according to this main chemical group (ester, phenol, ketone, aldehyde, and so on).

Although an essential oil is categorized according to its main group, it does not necessarily carry the properties of that main chemical group. Since an essential oil may contain several multicarbon compounds from different chemical groups, its therapeutic properties will depend on each of those groups. The influence of one chemical group on another, which is known as synergy, contributes specific therapeutic properties to each essential oil. More often than not, an essential oil has very different properties from those of its main chemical group. Furthermore, essential oils with the same main group will have different therapeutic properties from each other. The following example illustrates how three essential oils with the same main chemical group (ester) have completely different therapeutic properties.

The Synergy of Multicarbon Compounds

Three essential oils with the same main group but with different therapeutic properties.

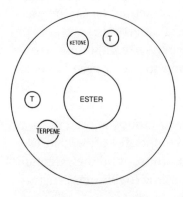

Chamaemelum nobile
(Roman chamomile)
Strong antispasmodic, especially
for the urogenital system.

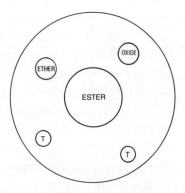

Laurus nobilis
(bay leaf)
Strong infection fighter.
Antispasmodic for the lungs.
General tonic.

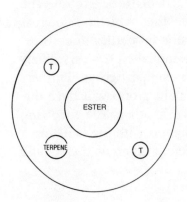

Citrus aurantium
(orange leaves)
Bactericidal and calming to the skin.

The examples show how difficult it is to determine which therapeutic effects an essential oil will have. Even if you have a chromatographic analysis of an essential oil and are familiar with the chemical properties of each group, a list of these properties would not describe the therapeutic action of the essential oil. An essential oil is like an individual, with a unique character, and it is a living molecule that is very active. For this reason, *essential oils are difficult to use and must be carefully administered by persons who have working knowledge of and experience with essential oils.*

Apart from its chemical specificity, it is thought that an essential oil can be organ-specific. Treatments given at the Institute of Biomedical and Philosophical Studies in France have given strong evidence for this belief. However, there are as yet no scientific studies establishing why an essential oil may be organ-specific—only clinical observations.

For example, the specific action of the immune response is a complicated process, involving the antibody's amino acid sequence. The same specificity can exist between a remedy, like an essential oil, and organ cells of the human body—if the energy patterns are identical. Perhaps essential oils that are specific to organs must contain molecules with energy patterns identical to those of the cells grouped in an organ. The uses of certain essential oils and how organ-specific they may be are discussed in more detail below.

An essential oil should be an undiluted plant product. It is important when purchasing such an oil to look for the label "Guaranteed 100% pure." This label ensures that the bottle is filled only with undiluted essential oil. The words "botanically certified" guarantee that the essential oil is either distilled from organically grown plants or has been analyzed for contaminants. This is important, since some essential oils are extracted from wild plants grown where pollutants may have contaminated soil and water.

Essential oils transfer their properties to the body via the bloodstream. They can enter the bloodstream three ways: by ingestion, by inhalation, and by application to the skin.

INGESTING ESSENTIAL OILS SAFELY AND EFFECTIVELY

Essential oils must be properly administered. They cannot be ingested in their pure form, but must be mixed with a neutral ingredient known as a vehicle. Since an essential oil is a pure, undiluted substance, it is extremely concentrated. To consume an essential oil as an oral remedy, one should mix it with honey—preferably unpasteurized. *Honey provides a vehicle that allows the essential oil to maintain its action without altering its chemical components. It also prevents irritation of the patient's mouth, throat, and stomach linings.* In addition, combining an essential oil with honey makes it easy to mix a batch of a prescribed remedy to be taken over a week. Essential oils can also be dropped on sugar cubes and the cube eaten like a candy. Although this provides a quick and easy way of consuming essential oils, unpasteurized honey is a better vehicle.

Aromatherapists will recommend a dosage of a certain number of drops of essential oil mixed in one cup of honey. Because pure, unpasteurized honey often has a hard consistency, it is a good idea to melt the honey by placing its glass container in hot water to facilitate mixing. Always use stainless steel utensils and glass containers when mixing essential oils. Wood and plastic absorb the oils.

Essential oils are bottled in colored glass so that they will not be oxidized by sun or other light sources. Keep any essential oil–honey mixture in a sealed container (a sterilized jar is ideal) and store it in a cool, dark place. Allowing an essential oil–honey mixture to sit for a week or two will permit greater distribution of the essential oil's energy and yield an all-round more homogenous mixture. When preparing a mixture ahead of time, slowly stir the mixture once a day for a week. *An essential oil–honey mixture stored in a cool, dark place can last indefinitely.*

According to a practicing aromatherapist, drinking a glass of warm water after consuming the essential-oil mixture in the dosage prescribed by the specialist or aromatherapist (usually 1 teaspoonful three times a day) helps disperse the honey mixture.

INHALING ESSENTIAL OILS

Inhalation is the only way to use pure essential oils undiluted with a vehicle. This can be done by simply applying a few drops of the essential oil on a handkerchief and breathing normally into the handkerchief. Or it can be done through vaporization. Dropping essential oils into a vaporizer or cool-mist humidifier will disperse the molecules of essential oil into the air. *Ambient air can be disinfected by applying certain essential oils to the vacuum cleaner filter just before vacuuming.* The essential oil will be dispersed through the vacuum's exhaust air. Essential oils can also be dropped into humidifiers. Diffusers especially made for essential oils use air pumps or nebulizers, which shoot a calibrated dose of liquid as a fine mist, sending the essential oil into the atmosphere without heating or altering it. These devices are useful for inhalation therapy as well as for disinfecting ambient air. They send pure essential-oil molecules into the air in your home, allowing the inhabitants to breathe these molecules. When candles made with essential oils incorporated into the wax are burned, they release oil's molecules into the air.

APPLYING ESSENTIAL OILS TO THE SKIN

Applying essential oils to the skin requires that they be diluted in an appropriate vehicle; since they are so concentrated, only a few drops are needed, but it is often impossible to cover the skin with only the necessary few drops. The appropriate vehicle for topical application of essential oils is vegetable or nut oil. Cold-pressed or virgin oils are preferred, because refined oils will rob the essential oil of its therapeutic properties. *Almond, safflower, saffron, and hazelnut oil are choice vehicles for applying essential oils to the skin.* You can use sesame oil, but some heavier essential oils, such as sandlewood, do not mix well and the essential oils will irritate your skin. An oil base is often avoided when essential oils are used for a rash or fungus infection because oils tend to clog pores, something you wish to avoid in fungal rashes. On small areas the undiluted essential oil can sometimes be used, if prescribed by a specialist. When greater coverage with a nonoily vehicle is required, aloe vera juice or gel can be used. Aloe vera seems to enhance the properties of the essential oils. In addition, aloe vera has been shown to have its own therapeutic properties, which are mostly beneficial in treating skin conditions. In test cases, aloe vera performed as well as or better than the recommended prescription drugs. Aloe vera penetrates the skin efficiently and does not leave a film. Applied topically, essential oils penetrate the skin quickly, and most descend to the basal layer of the skin, known as the vascular tissue, which is packed with blood vessels. At this level, essential oils begin to actively change the biochemical canvas of the skin through subtle biochemical reactions and changes in energy patterns.

When essential oils are mixed with aloe vera, they can be prepared ahead of time, if kept in sealed glass containers and stored in cold, dark locations. A 99.6 percent solution of aloe vera should be used. Juices or gels that do not indicate the percentage of aloe vera may not be extracted from mature plants and thus may not have the therapeutic benefits associated with a pure extract. A solution of 99.6 percent or higher must be pure and not contain such additives as potassium sorbate. Additives often cause skin irritations and so would oppose the treatment. A good solution of aloe vera will contain natural preservatives like Irish moss and vitamin C—substances that are compatible with essential oils. *A mixture of essential oils and aloe vera can be applied to large surface areas with a mister.* Unlike honey or oil solutions, aloe vera mixtures prepared ahead of time will only keep for two to three weeks. If there is a change in odor, the mixture must be discarded and a new batch made.

Essential oils do *not* mix with water. Dropping essential oils into a glass of water or juice, or into the bathtub, is like dropping a match into a bathtub full of water. The essential oil's action is nullified. Moreover, certain essential oils are dermocaustic, chemically burning the skin. These essential oils stay on the surface of the bath water, where they can come in direct contact with the skin, burning it and leaving a difficult-to-remove damaging film.

Certain methods of administration are inappropriate with some essential oils. One example is essential oil of lavender. This oil loses 90 percent of its properties if it is used as an oral remedy and is best used as an inhalant or on the skin. Other essential oils, such as cedar leaf, are used as repellents or domestic disinfectants, since they contain highly toxic chemical groups.

The chemical specificity of essential oils imposes many restraints on their use. These remedies can work wonders, but they must be administered by a specialist—an aromatherapist who is well versed in the chemical specificity. Unfortunately, people who are experienced with the uses of essential oils are rare. In the past, most of the information dealing with the clinical uses of essential oils came from Europe. And although many of the studies were conducted under controlled conditions, they were never published in scientific journals but rather were passed on to the holistic medical community by means of professional conferences and seminars. Recently, North America has discovered the beneficial clinical applications of essential oils, and close to a dozen articles about them have been published in American scientific journals. At the University of Wisconsin *researchers have discovered that essential oil of orange peel can prevent the formation of mammary tumors and reduce preformed cancerous tumors. Further investigation has given convincing evidence that essential oil of orange strengthens the immune system.* This research was published in the *Journal of the National Cancer In-*

stitute in 1986, and in *Carcinogenesis* in 1988. Maltzman's study, reported in *The Federation Proceedings*, 1986, revealed that the essential oil of orange peel was more effective than the isolated terpene d-limonene. This study supports the holistic principle that each part of the whole biosystem contributes properties that are transferred to the body when the remedy is ingested. The isolated compound, in contrast, only carries part of the energy and properties of its original biosystem.

DOSAGE

There is only one rule to follow when using essential oils. They must be used in minute doses. *The old adage "if a little is good, a lot is better" does not apply to essential oils.* Many essential oils with a high concentration of phenol are dangerous, and a high dosage can reverse their therapeutic effects. The use of essential oils in small doses (by the drop) does not only apply to essence taken internally. Some essential oils irritate the skin and must not be used on the skin or in the bath. Essential oils are completely compatible with, and often act as adjuvants with, herbal remedies (herb capsules, tinctures, extracts), but they may be contraindicated with homeopathic remedies. Since the chemical composition of an essential oil is so specific, therapy must be left to a professional. Unfortunately, most allopathic physicians, and many homeopaths and naturopaths, are not entirely familiar with essential oils. Specialists working clinically and researching these substances make themselves available to doctors and can be approached for guidance. Often, by contacting a manufacturer of essential oils, you can be referred to either a researcher or an experienced aromatherapist. When you are searching for these specialists, it is important to seek advice from the manufacturers, and not the distributors. Although essential oils are sold in health food stores, their personnel is not a competent source of information, especially about essential oils. However, these stores do carry books on related subjects, and sometimes the names of professionals who can provide guidance.

Organic essential oils can be extremely beneficial when placed in the right hands, but they can be exceedingly dangerous when used by unqualified, uninformed individuals.

USEFUL ESSENTIAL OILS

It is impossible to describe every essential oil here, but since essential oils are available without prescription, there are a few that should be familiar to everyone. Lavender and rosemary are particularly beneficial, and these standard essences should be included in the holistic medicine cabinet.

Essential Oil of Lavender

There are several species of lavender. True lavender *(Lavandula vera)* contains coumarin—a fragrant inorganic substance that prolongs distillation of the essential oil and makes it costly. This is the main reason why the commercially available essential oil of lavender is usually derived from *Lavandula spica,* a domestic species of lavender.

Lavandula spica

Lavandula spica contains an oxide and a ketone in almost equal proportion, as well as small amounts of terpenes. The synergy of these chemical groups contributes the following properties to *Lavandula spica:*
—It kills germs.
—It is a decongestant, especially for the breathing passages and lungs.
—It is an expectorant.

Lavandula spica is recommended as:
1. An inhalant—using a few drops on a handkerchief—for colds and for congestion due to allergy.

2. A topical remedy, pure or mixed with cold-pressed vegetable oil, to produce an effective rub for rheumatic pain.
Applied in its pure form to areas of the skin where there is
neuralgia, headache, toothache, or menstrual cramps, and
to fungal infections, like athlete's foot, to minor burns, and
to skin irritations due to bacterial infections or acne.

Lavandula vera

True lavender, or *Lavandula vera,* is sometimes found commercially as an essential oil. The plants distilled are wild, so it is important to make sure that the product comes from a reputable
company that guarantees that the essential oil has been batch-
tested for contaminants, with the words "100% guaranteed
pure and botanically certified" inscribed on the label.

Lavandula vera contains a high concentration of an ester. It
contains ketones, coumarins, oxides, and terpenes in similar
proportion, and a good proportion of alcohols. The synergy of
these chemicals gives *Lavandula vera* its properties. It is:
—An anti-inflammatory
—An anticoagulant
—An antispasmodic
—A sedative
—Germicidal
—A decongestant, for broncho-pulmonary and circulatory sys-
tems

It is recommended as:
1. An inhalant to decongest stuffy nose and congestion due to
colds and allergy. *As an inhalant,* Lavandula vera *will kill
many bacterial forms and some viruses infecting the breathing
passages. It also contributes a calming effect.*
2. A topical remedy, pure or mixed with a cold-pressed vegetable oil to form a rub to increase circulation (especially venous flow), and to relieve pain from neuralgia, muscle

spasms from injury and fatigue, and menstrual pain. This mixture may also be used for a relaxing bath. It may be applied pure to skin irritations due to allergy, burns, or ulcers and to cuts and abrasions.

3. Neither variety of lavender should be consumed internally, not because they are dangerous, but because they are more effective when applied topically or used as inhalants.

Lavandula vera is a gem of an essential oil. If a specialist is lucky enough to find it, it should be carefully preserved.

All essential oils of lavender may be used in a diffuser or vacuum cleaner to freshen and disinfect the air. They may also be used as a topical disinfectant for minor cuts and scrapes and as an anti-inflammatory for bruises and sprains and for minor burns.

Essential Oil of Rosemary

True Rosemary

Several species of rosemary are used for essential oils. True rosemary *(Rosmarinus officinalis)* contains almost equal proportions of a ketone and an ester, a fair amount of an oxide and some terpenes and alcohols. The synergy of these chemical groups gives *Rosmarinus officinalis* its properties. It is:

−A blood purifier; especially effective in flushing cholesterol
−A liver decongestant
−A circulatory aid
−A general stimulant
−An antispasmodic
−An antidepressant, or anxiety fighter
−A tonic

It is generally recommended as:

1. An oral remedy to purify blood. As a blood purifier, dislodging waxy buildup of cholesterol and stimulating the circula-

tory system. It can be useful in treating the buildup of allo-pathic drugs, foods, and preservatives. It is an adjuvant to certain vitamin therapy.

2. An oral remedy for liver ailments, particularly slow or le-thargic liver. True rosemary stimulates the organs, specific-ally the liver. It decongests engorged livers and stimulates the gallbladder to secrete bile. It can be useful in certain kid-ney infections.

3. An oral remedy for spasms of organs and systems, particu-larly the cardiovascular system, with some effect on the lungs. It relaxes soft-tissue muscles by regulating blood flow.

4. An oral remedy that regulates and stimulates body func-tions, particularly at the organ level. *By regulating body functions, true rosemary prevents physiological stress and therefore fights anxiety.* Its action as a general stimulant makes true rosemary a tonic; by stimulating body functions, it supports such processes as digestion, elimination, oxygenation, and neurotransmission.

True rosemary grows wild in Provence, France, as well as in other mountainous areas of Europe. Labels must indicate the area where the plants have been harvested, and because the plants distilled are wild, the certification "100% guaranteed pure and botanically certified" ensures that they have been batch-tested for contaminants.

Cultivated Rosemary

Essential oil of cultivated rosemary (also *Rosmarinus officinalis*) is earmarked as an oxide because of its high concentration of this chemical group. It also contains a fair amount of ketones and small amounts of terpenes and alcohols. The synergy of these chemicals gives cultivated rosemary the following properties:

—It is a decongestant and is mucinolytic, especially for the broncho-pulmonary system and the circulatory system.
—It is slightly germicidal.

It is recommended as:
1. An oral remedy for cough and pulmonary congestion due to colds, allergy, or infection. It is excellent for thinning mucous secretions. It stimulates circulation, thus helping to relieve edema of circulatory ailments due to poor nutrition, injury, or genetic predisposition to rheumatic or arthritic conditions.
2. An oral remedy effective in killing certain types of bacteria and viruses. It is more effective in this capacity, however, when combined with other essential oils.

Mediterranean Rosemary

Wild rosemary harvested in Mediterranean regions contains a large proportion of ketone and has the characteristic odor of camphor. It also contains an oxide and an ester in almost equal proportion, as well as some alcohols and terpenes. The synergy of these chemical groups gives rosemary grown in Mediterranean regions its properties. It is:
−A tonic, especially for the cardiovascular system
−A decongestant for the circulatory system (venous flow)
−A muscle relaxant
−Mucinolytic
−Germicidal
−Anti-inflammatory

It is recommended as:
1. An oral remedy for certain heart conditions. In minute doses (always prescribed by physicians), it can lower blood pressure.
2. An oral remedy for circulatory problems due to heart conditions affecting venous flow. Also useful in the treatment of varicose veins.
3. A topical remedy in the form of a massage oil to relax tired, injured, and stressed muscles.
4. A topical remedy for toothache and headache.

5. An oral remedy for coughs.
6. An oral remedy for certain infections when combined with other essential oils.

Mediterranean rosemary is dangerous and should never be taken by those with high blood pressure unless at a physician's advice. Even normal doses can cause high blood pressure in susceptible people. Incorrect doses can cause altered properties that can be very dangerous, even toxic. When there is no identification on the bottle indicating where the plants were cultivated, the distinct smell of camphor will identify the essential oil as Mediterranean rosemary. Although each type of essential oil of rosemary has a slight odor of camphor, Mediterranean rosemary smells exclusively of camphor.

Essential Oil of Clove

This is a dangerous essential oil because of its high concentration of phenol. *Essential oil of clove* (**Syzqium Aromaticum**) *must* not *be administered to pregnant women or animals, since it causes dilation of the uterus, which can lead to miscarriage or abortion.* Essential oil of clove can destroy certain viruses, bacteria, and parasites. Properly prescribed, it is extremely beneficial in the treatment of certain viruses and is a potent anthelmintic (worming) medicine.

It is recommended as:
1. An oral remedy, *under prescription,* for viral infections and expulsion of parasites.
2. A topical remedy mixed in very minute amounts with vegetable oils or vitamin E to produce a phenolic oil that helps remove the crusts formed by eczema.

Essential Oil of Chamomile

Roman Chamomile

Two essential oils of chamomile are available commercially. The more common oil is derived from Roman chamomile *(Chamaemelum nobile)* and contains an ester and a ketone in almost equal proportion. It is a potent antispasmodic and has some anticoagulant properties. It is a tonic for the nervous system and lowers fever.

It is recommended as an oral remedy in the treatment of digestive, urinary tract, and urogenital tract ailments. Because of its anticoagulant and sedative properties, it is useful in appeasing menstrual cramps and can help relieve symptoms of PMS (premenstrual syndrome) and menopause.

German Chamomile

The second essential oil of chamomile is derived from German chamomile *(Matricartita chamomilla)* and has the characteristic blue tint of azulene, a terpene used in many cosmetics as an anti-inflammatory agent. The properties of this essential oil are very different from those of Roman chamomile.

German chamomile is recommended as a topical remedy for the treatment of skin irritations, and cosmetically for sensitive skin.

Essential Oil of Marjoram

Essential oil of marjoram *(Origanum marjorana)* has a high concentration of alcohols, and a fair amount of esters, with some terpenes. The synergy of these chemicals makes it quite versatile. It is a general tonic, stimulates digestion, and is antispasmodic, especially for the digestive tract. It is analgesic and anti-inflammatory, especially when applied topically.

It is recommended as:

1. An oral remedy in treating digestive disturbances. It is a general stimulant that can be used as an adjuvant in the treatment of debilitating diseases and chronic fatigue and lethargy. It is a good general tonic during convalescence.
2. A topical rub combined with other essential oils to relieve pain and inflammation of sprains, rheumatism, and stressed muscles.

Essential Oil of Wild Carrot

Essential oil of wild carrot *(Daucus carota)* is distilled from the seeds of the wild carrot plant that grows wild in fields, usually in the Mediterranean basin. The characteristic spray of purple pigment in the middle of each white flower distinguishes this plant from the toxic Aethusa *(Aethusa cynapium)* plant. *The distillation of essential oil of wild carrot is delicate, and thus it is especially important to obtain this substance from a reputable company.* Wild carrot's essential oil is unique in containing several chemical groups in almost equal proportion. It is earmarked as a terpene because of the high concentration of this group.

It is recommended as:

1. An oral remedy for the treatment of liver ailments. It stimulates and "cleans" the liver.
2. An oral remedy for anemia. Clinical studies at the Institute of Biomedical and Philosophical Studies in France indicate that consumption of essential oil of carrot increases the level of hemoglobin, an iron-containing substance found in red blood cells that picks up oxygen and carries it to organs. Thus essential oil of carrot is considered to help in the treatment and prevention of anemia.
3. An oral remedy to help fight high cholesterol and diabetes. Studies by the institute also indicate that this substance is

useful in the treatment and prevention of diabetes and that it reduces the level of cholesterol.

4. An oral remedy for cardiac conditions. Given in proper proportion, wild carrot's essential oil can regulate the heart rate and reduce cardiac edema by regulating blood flow through the cardiac system.
5. A topical remedy. Essential oil of wild carrot regenerates skin cells. Applied pure or mixed with cold-pressed vegetable oils, it is useful in treating skin conditions caused by sun and wind damage, skin eruptions due to poor nutrition, chapped, cracked skin, and nonmalignant skin tumors. It is also helpful in treating eczema.

Essential Oil of Bay Leaf

Essential oil of bay leaf *(Laurus nobilis)* contains equal proportions of esters and oxides. It also contains some terpenes, alcohols, and a small amount of phenols. This essential oil is very active.

It is recommended as:
1. An oral remedy to fight infections, particularly of the broncho-pulmonary area, making it useful in treating colds and flu.
2. An oral antispasmodic remedy for the lungs and a potent expectorant.
3. An oral remedy as a general tonic and stimulant. It has mild action on the nervous system, especially brain function.
4. An oral remedy to fight infection by stimulating the immune system. It is often used as an oral remedy to stimulate body functions (because it seems to have a stimulating action on all body systems) in cases of chronic fatigue, debilitating illnesses, infections, and old age. *Essential oil of bay leaf is a potent tonic for the elderly.*

Essential Oil of Peppermint

Essential oil of peppermint *(Mentha piperita)* has a high concentration of ketones and alcohols, a few esters and oxides, and some terpenes. The chemical composition of this essential oil varies according to the area where the plant source grew.

Doses of this essential oil must be exact, since it behaves differently in different doses. In high doses, it can become a dangerous convulsive. In low doses, it can be a digestive antispasmodic and relieve intestinal gas. It can stimulate the liver and relieve nausea, and but in some individuals it will cause nausea and headache. Peppermint stimulates brain activity. When essence of peppermint was piped into the ventilation system in factories in China, worker productivity increased. As an inhalant or an oral remedy, essential oil of peppermint can relieve fatigue and lethargy, but it can cause headaches and high blood pressure in sensitive individuals if doses are not accurate.

It is recommended as:
1. An inhalant to relieve fatigue and lethargy.
2. An oral remedy (in accurate doses) to relieve fatigue and lethargy and intestinal gas.
3. An oral antiworm remedy, which will also regulate intestinal flora, especially after convalescence or drug therapy and particularly with antibiotics.
4. An oral remedy to fight infection; usually used in combination with other essential oils.

Although all these essential oils are useful, they should not be used in self-treatment. They are described only to give you a better understanding of these remedies. Armed with facts, one is better able to participate in medical treatment, rather than passively turning over one's body, mind, and spirit to a health professional.

FOR FURTHER READING

Clegg, R. J.; Middleton, B.; Bell, G. D.; and White, D. A. "Inhibition of Hepatic Cholesteral Synthesis by Monoterpenes Administered in Vivo," *Biochemical Pharmacology* 29 (1980).

Evans, D.; Miller, D.; Jacobsen, K.: and Bush, P. "Modulation of Immune Responses in Mice by D-limonene." *Journal of Toxicological and Environmental Health* 20 (1987).

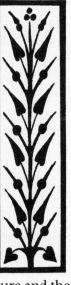

SEVEN

Herb and Other Plant Preparations

This chapter focuses on remedies made from herbs and plants, outlining their manufacture and the uses of the different types of products. Although the therapeutic action of individual herbs is not discussed, because of the huge scope of the subjects, many books on this topic are available (see the readings at the end of this chapter).

A herb is a plant that is usually aromatic and is used in cooking or in medicine. A herb is usually fleshy, like grass, without any apparent woody parts. In this chapter, the word "plant" will refer to both herbs and nonherb plants.

Healing with the products of nature was the genesis of medicine and remedies. The therapeutic use of plants has existed among the most ancient civilizations of the world. These ancient practices and the records of substances and their observed therapeutic values have given us modern-day treatments with herbs, as well as allopathic drugs.

All drugs of the past were substances with a particular therapeutic action extracted from plants. With the evolution of technology, extraction processes could be replaced by synthesis in laboratory. But the synthetic duplication of the molecules found in nature changes the overall action of the drug in the body.

As explained earlier, drugs have a problematic biphasic effect, whereas whole herbs do not. Extraction of a herb's active principle will alter the biochemical and bioenergetic action of that substance because the integrated substances in the biosystem are lost. Fragmenting the plant's biosystem by extraction of only the active principles limits and changes the effects of the individual substances.

This is not to say that fragmentation of medicinal plants does not have its place. A new technology in the bioengineering of new molecules from plant substances is an important step in medicine. Instead of creating synthetic drugs that cause deterioration of the body, bioengineers are creating complex substances from plant biosystems. These substances are specific to diseases and also restore the body's natural "healing sense." Unfortunately, these medicines are only selectively available at this time, and are extremely expensive to produce; therefore, they are used mostly by physician-researchers in clinical research.

It is much cheaper to copy nature in the laboratory than to harvest its benefits through extraction procedures—hence, the deviation that took place between natural remedies and drugs. *The separation of holistic and allopathic medicine was an economic phenomenon, based on the evolution of society through industry rather than on the advancement of medicine and the evolution of a healthy society.* Today we can clearly see the results of such a perspective. In the inevitable cycle of nature, the progression of industry leads us right back to "natural" methods. Now we need remedies to prevent and treat the diseases that have occurred as a result of the spoils of industry, such as those linked to pollution. Although the division between natural and allopathic remedies still exists today, scientific research and investigation are being conducted on the effects of such natural remedies as vitamins and minerals, herbal tinctures, herbal preparations, homeopathic remedies, and Chinese herbs.

WHY ARE HERBS THERAPEUTIC?

Essentially all plants have therapeutic properties because all plants contain a variety of biologically active substances. All plants undergo photosynthesis, which uses the sun's energy to transform carbon dioxide from the atmosphere into energy-rich substances, like sugars. The carbon chains resulting from photosynthesis are further transformed into a variety of types of compounds, like lipids, alkaloids, essential oils, and tannins. And through other biochemical processes, minerals and nitrates absorbed by the roots from the soil are transformed into vitamins, trace minerals, and antibiotics.

Herbs can affect biological systems at the cell and organ level. Although they do contribute the energy of their original biostate, they do not act at an entirely energetic level, as do homeopathic herbal dilutions. Taking herbs can lead to high blood levels of biologically active substances, which can produce pharmacological and therapeutic effects.

Heterocyclic Compounds

A heterocyclic compound is a cyclic molecule in which the ring contains more than one kind of element. Natural heterocyclic compounds include chlorophyll (the plant pigment involved in photosynthesis), hemoglobin (which gives blood its red color), and sugars. Heterocyclic compounds are formed by complex processes that vary from plant to plant. They range from poisons, like strychnine, to such healing agents as digitalis, a heart tonic derived from the foxglove *(Digitalis purpurea)* plant.

Alkaloids

Alkaloids are complex plant molecules, many with powerful poisoning activity. They are found in different parts of plants. For example, morphine is an alkaloid found in the fruit of the

poppy, and quinine is found in the bark of cinchona. It is estimated that 15 to 20 percent of flowering plants contain alkaloids. *Some alkaloids are used as medicinal drugs. In even infinitesimal amounts, they function with biochemical precision.*

Tannins

These substances give a brownish color to plants. They are considered to be the by-products of the plant's metabolism. Tannins
are very common in plants and can make up as much as 20 percent of a plant's weight. In medicine, tannins are used as astringents and to counter the effects of certain poisons.

Antibiotics

Many plants manufacture antibiotics. Certain sulfur-containing
compounds from garlic provide examples of these. Mustard contains a heterocyclic compound that is antibiotic in nature.

WHICH PARTS OF A PLANT ARE THERAPEUTIC?

Active substances are unequally distributed throughout a plant.
The leaves, which are the site of photosynthesis, contain most of
the heterocyclic compounds, as well as the alkaloids. Since these
substances are the active ingredients of many remedies and
drugs, the leaves of a plant are most frequently used for teas and
other preparations derived from dried plants. The stems are the
highways for the chemical substances that circulate through
plants, and under optimal conditions, certain active ingredients
may be present in the stem; this plant part is not commonly used
in herbal preparations, however. Often the sapwood contains
active substances. The bark also is used for herbal preparations.
Buds may contain antiseptic substances. Rhizomes, tubers, and
bulbs contain minerals, vitamins, antibiotics, and nutrients like
sugar and starch that sustain the plant through the winter. The

roots too may contain sugars, but they are known for their high concentration of minerals, which they draw from the soil and pump to the others parts of the plant. Certain species, under certain conditions, may have alkaloids in their roots. The flowers contain the reproductive material of the plant, as well as essential oils and pigments that color the petals. Flowers also contain substances called flavonoids, which are yellow organic molecules from the chemical ketone group. The fruit and stems of fruit are rich in vitamins and minerals, and may contain sulfurous substances, organic acids, and sugars. The seeds contain nutrients essential to the growth of the plant, such as lipids and sugars, as well as starches and vegetable oils.

Other medicines may be derived from secretions of the plant. Resin and gums are often used in poultices used to draw out pus from abscesses.

EACH PLANT PART HAS A BOILING TIME

The plant part used in the preparation of teas or infusions from dried herbs is of particular importance. Apart from the active principles contained within each part, attention must be given to handling of the particular plant part. For example, heat from boiled water may destroy certain active principles. To reap the benefits of the ingredients contained in each part of the plant, careful consideration must be given to the boiling time of each part. *In general, the boiling or steeping time decreases as you go up the plant.* For instance, flowers should be steeped for not more than 2 minutes. Intense steeping will not make a stronger infusion but will destroy many of the flower's active ingredients. Leaves and stems may be steeped for 5 to 10 minutes. Roots and bark should be thrown into boiling water and simmered for 3 to 7 minutes, until the water turns to a rich color—usually brown or gold.

As discussed in previous chapters, the active ingredients contained in a plant depend on many factors:

1. Geographical location of the plant
   −Traditionally, plants grown in the wild have a greater concentration of active principles than those grown in hothouses under controlled environmental conditions. Latitude is particularly important, and plants grown in mountainous regions usually have great medicinal value.
2. The weather
   −Plants grown in areas of rough weather, parching winds, and drought will have a higher concentration of essential oils as well as other active ingredients.
3. Soil
   −The mineral content of plants depends on the soil.
4. Life stage of the plant
   − *In most cases, mature plants yield greater concentrations of active substances than young plants do.* These active substances undergo radical chemical changes during flowering and a plant may contain ingredients during flowering that it does not contain out of season. The chemicals found in a dried herb will depend on the time when the fresh plant was harvested.
5. Part of the plant used
   −Different plant parts contain different substances.

All these factors are interrelated. Together they influence the chemical composition of a plant.

DRYING PROCEDURES

Air-Drying

Plants are usually separated into their respective parts as soon as they have been picked. This is an important step, because if plants are store whole, chemical reactions may occur, changing the ingredients sought from one part or another. The separated parts are placed on racks that allow air to circulate over and under them. Each rack holds the same plant parts; that is, all the leaves are placed on one rack, all the stems are placed on another rack, and so on. Racks are usually made of stainless steel, since other metals and plastic may cause reactions or leaching of the plant elements.

Some manufacturers wash plants after they are picked, whereas others wash them after they have been separated. After the plants have been washed, they are blasted with hot or warm air. Since root fragments dry more quickly and efficiently than the whole root, which may putrefy, roots are then cut into pieces measuring about two centimetres. The plant parts undergo drying in special chambers that either have natural air circulation or mechanized circulation. Whichever it is, the air flow is a gentle one. The chamber must be dark to prevent any chemical changes of the active principles of the plant due to light. Commercial chambers are sterile, with elaborate air filtration systems to prevent dust and pollen contamination. Some European drying chambers are made of stainless steel to prevent any kind of oxidation reactions within the plants.

Some herbalists leave the plants in the sun for about two hours after they have been separated into parts, but commercial enterprises rarely do this. In fact, *it is better for the plant to be uniformly dried rather than undergo the temperature change caused by exposure to sunlight*. Moreover, oxidation reactions have been associated with ultraviolet light. Oxidation reactions cause alteration or destruction of chemicals and yield free radicals, which damage the cell tissues of the body (see chapter 11). Every day the plants, or sometimes the racks, are gently turned to favor uniform drying.

Drying removes between 75 and 85 percent of the plants' water. Aquatic plants lose up to 90 percent of their water content during drying. The season of harvest also plays a role in how much water a plant will lose during drying. Plants picked during the spring will lose more water than those harvested in the fall. Optimum drying procedures leave 10 to 12 percent water. This is important, as it maintains the chemical composition of a plant, as well as its energy imprint.

Water can be charged with various types of energies. Several experiments showing the capacity of water to "hold" energies have been verified by scientists around the world. For this reason, plants that are grown in polluted environments can pick up detrimental energy patterns as a result of pollutants in water.

During drying, different plant species are never mixed, for this could cause reactions that would change the chemistry of the dried plants. Drying time depends on the species and size of the plant and on how much water will be removed. Once plants have been dried, they are packaged, usually in plastic or cellophane bags, labeled, and sold. Herbs that go into capsules are ground and capsulized. Plants used in tea bags are minced and bagged.

Freeze-Drying

"Lyophilization" is the technical term for freeze-drying. During freeze-drying, water is removed from frozen material by a chemical process known as sublimation. This process allows the active ingredients contained within plant materials to become trapped as solid particles, preserving the chemical nature of the active principles. Enzymes are also inactivated during this process but not destroyed. The volatile substances, such as the essential oils, are susceptible to most commercial processing and are often destroyed. Freeze-drying prevents the destruction of these substances. In chapter 3 you saw that active principles are soluble in alcohol, but alcohol can remove certain important plant components, such as polysaccharides, by precipitation. Furthermore, with the removal of most of the water during freeze-drying, there is not enough moisture left to promote enzymatic activity, which may change the chemical nature of a product during storage. A low level of moisture prevents the growth of mold and bacteria, an important factor, since bacteria alter substances by causing the fermentation of sugars. Reduced moisture also slows down the degradation of plant pigments such a chlorophyll and water-soluble vitamins. Furthermore, the low-temperature process minimizes the rate of biochemical reactions, since fewer chemical reactions occur at low temperatures.

Basically, freeze-drying involves:

– The freezing of plant material by low-temperature cooling.
– The drying of frozen material by direct sublimation at reduced pressure.
– The storage in airtight, opaque containers of the freeze-dried material.

The freeze-drying of herbs has become highly sophisticated. It stabilizes and preserves active principles, inhibits growth of microorganisms and degeneration of the product, and prolongs shelf life.

Freeze-drying is expensive and in the past was reserved for medical pharmaceuticals such as plasma, vaccines, sera, spermatozoa, and skin and bone grafts. Making and purchasing freeze-dried herbs is well worth the expense, though, for it yields a better, more complete product. In fact, *the freeze-dried herb is biochemically identical to its fresh state*. This means that not only are the active components of the plant preserved unaltered, but the energy pattern of the plant cells is also maintained, giving a product that is most compatible with the body. In a sense, a lyophilized herb is a suspended biosystem that will be reanimated once consumed by another biosystem.

REMEDIES TO MAKE WITH DRIED HERBS, AND THEIR USES

Dried plants are probably the most versatile elements used in natural remedies. Herbal preparations prepared at home are economical. But often air-dried herbs lose their therapeutic properties because their active principles are destroyed by heat, air, or sunlight. Although dried herbs can be kept indefinitely if stored in dark, sealed containers, once they are rehydrated with a liquid, these home-dried herbs may not be as therapeutic as

commercially available ones. Herbal preparations apply to almost any health situation.

Teas

Teas are prepared by steeping the dried plant(s) in water. There
are three different types of tea preparations: infusions, decoctions, and macerations.

Infusions

Infusions are prepared by pouring boiling water over specific
plant parts, usually flowers. These should steep for 2 minutes.
When the leaves are used, the mixture can steep for up to 10
minutes. *Infusions should be prepared in a glazed enamel container,
preferably with a cover to conserve the steam, which contains many
volatile substances that have a therapeutic nature.* Drink the infusion as soon as possible to prevent the active elements from
being destroyed by heat or escaping through the vapor. An infusion made with mullein *(Verbascum thapsus)* flowers is a European favorite for respiratory complaints such as bronchitis.

Decoctions

A decoction involves placing dried plants in cold water, and
bringing the mixture to the boiling point, and allowing it to boil
about 5 minutes (sometimes 10 for certain roots) in a closed
container. This solution is often used for skin applications, as in
the European tradition of washing cuts and abrasions with a decoction made of lavender *(Lavandula vera)*. A bouillon consists
of a decoction using the whole plant, and is consumed like soup.
The boiling time of a bouillon varies with the species of plant.

Macerations

A home-made maceration involves soaking dried plants in water, wine, or alcohol for several days, or sometimes weeks. The

mixture is kept in a closed container in a cool (not refrigerated), dark place. The resulting mixture is very strong, containing a high concentration of active principles. A maceration has considerable therapeutic value. A maceration made from valerian *(Valeriana officinalis)* roots is an interesting French remedy for reducing appetite.

Inhalations

Aromatic plants are placed in hot water so that the patient may inhale the vapors that contain the volatile active ingredients of the plant. *An inhalation made from eucalyptus* **(Eucalyptus globulus)** *leaves is often recommended by naturopaths to relieve sinusitis.*

Poultices

A poultice is made by combining a decoction with medicinal clay. Generally, white or green clay is used for poultices rather than gray clay. Clays are inexpensive and are available at health food stores. A poultice is applied to the skin to draw out pus. Poultices are usually applied warm but may be used cold. In Europe a poultice made from geranium Robert *(Geranium robertianum)* leaves is applied to tender, painful breasts.

Wraps

A wrap, which is used for bandaging an ailing limb, is produced by soaking sterile gauze in a decoction. The wrap is always applied warm; the heat is part of the therapy. Sometimes the wrap is covered with a piece of plastic and a towel is placed over the plastic to conserve the heat. Naturopaths in Europe recommend wrapping sprains with a decoction of arnica *(Arnica montana)* leaves and flowers.

Baths and Washes

A bath involves immersing the entire body in a bath prepared from decoctions or infusions. These either compose the bath liquid or are mixed into the bath water. Washes are decoctions or infusions used locally to rinse the eyes, throat, or mouth. The Delaware Indians prepared a cold infusion from purple boneset *(Eupatorium purpureum)*, a wash they used for skin eruptions and irritations.

Liniments

Homemade liniments can be made by combining macerations with rubbing alcohol or oil. Many combinations of herbs are used to make liniments, which are used to stimulate circulation and thus warm or cool the injured or sore area. A popular European liniment combines peppermint leaves *(Mentha piperita)*, eucalyptus leaves *(Eucalyptus radiata)*, and rosemary leaves *(Rosmarinus officinalis)*.

Powders

Dried plants can be easily reduced to power with a mortar and pestle, or even a blender. Powders can be dusted on skin to treat external wounds. They can also be sprinkled on food or combined with water for hot or cold drinks. The Blackfoot Indians applied the dried powdered root of false Solomon's seal *(Smilacina racemosa)* to their skin to treat boils, sores, and wounds.

Syrups

Homemade syrup can be prepared by combining an infusion or a maceration with sugar and allowing the mixture to simmer until it thickens slightly. Brown sugar, honey, or treacle is the best choice for syrups, which are generally used as cough remedies. The Catawba Indians made a syrup from the boiled roots of mullein *(Verbascum thapsus)* as a cough remedy for children.

Saps

Sap is a natural product of plants and can be obtained by collecting the sap from the bark of trees with modern devices that screw into the tree trunk or by pressing the fruit or leaves. In the spring Europeans tap birch *(Betula alba)* and drink the resultant sap as a tonic. The Maine Penobscot Indians applied the gum of the balsam fir *(Abies balsamea)* to heal burns and sores. *The Kwakiutl Indians of British Columbia consumed the gum obtained from boiling juniper* (Juniperus communis) *berries to purify their blood and relieve shortness of breath.*

Wines

Wines are produced by soaking the bark, roots, or leaves or certain plants in wine. The plant parts should remain soaking in sealed containers and kept in a dark, cool place for at least three months. Renowned naturopath Dr. A. Vogel recommends rosemary *(Rosmarinus officinalis)* wine to speed recovery from the flu.

Elixirs

An elixir is used to invigorate the body by generally stimulating organ function. Commercial elixirs are prepared by first macerating fresh plants in alcohol and then distilling this solution. The resultant liquid is often mixed with sugar—either crude or refined—with honey, or with malt extract before it is bottled as an elixir. However, an elixir may be prepared from dried plants by soaking them in a mixture of alcohol and sugar. Red clover

(Trifolium pratense) is a common elixir in European folk medicine.

Other herbal preparations cannot be prepared at home but are made in the laboratory through specific chemical procedures. Some examples follow.

Extracts

Extracts are prepared by drying plants, separating them into parts, chopping or powdering them, and washing or percolating them with a solvent—water, alcohol, or ether. This process is called lixiviation. A common example of lixiviation is the making of coffee extract. Coffee beans are reduced to powder, then steam is forced through the coffee powder, and the resulting solution is evaporated to the desired concentration. Extracts are very potent herbal remedies. They are used extensively in clinical research, since they are one of the purest forms of herbal derivatives. Scientific studies have revealed that extract of echinacea *(Echinacea angustifolia)*, or purple cone flower, stimulates the immune system.

Tinctures

Refer to chapter 8 for details about tinctures. Tinctures are dried plants macerated in alcohol. They may also be obtained by lixiviation and percolation of alcohol. Generally, five parts alcohol are used for every equal part of dried herb. Tinctures are the most commonly available type of liquid herbal remedy. They are prepared from different herbs for different applications; for example, *naturopaths often recommend tincture of green anise* **(Pimpinella anisum)** *to relieve stomach cramps.*

Herbal Mixtures

As the name implies, herbal mixtures are combinations of plants. But for a herbal combination to be effective, it must be combined in the proper proportion with analogous herbs. In other words, there must be synergy. This is a combination in which the presence of one substance enhances the effects of another substance. In herbal mixtures, the therapeutic properties of all herbs combined must be the same—that is, antispasmodic, laxative, decongestant, and so on. The synergy of analogous herbs produces a "type" according to the main property of the herbs used in the mixture.

HERBS COMPARED WITH ALLOPATHIC DRUGS

Plants are living biosystems with their own energy imprint. The active principles in a plant are the therapeutic components of the plant—the natural drug. The action of these, within the plant's biosystem as well as within another biosystem (human or animal that consumes the plant), is influenced by other, apparently neutral components of the plant. Together the neutral components and the medicinal principles of the plant compose a "remedy," which can zero in on certain organs or systems of the body, altering the individual's energy pattern.

Allopathic drugs contribute only therapeutic properties. In most cases, they do not influence the energy pattern of the body but may negate healing energy by imposing the biphasic effect that turns the body against the healing treatment. In short, synthetic drugs are not biological complexes. Laboratory reproductions of plant-derived substances cannot copy the synergism of the naturally occurring plant substance or the energy imprint of the plant's biosystem.

This loss of properties also occurs with plant-derived substances when whole herbs are broken apart. In nature, molecules do not exist by themselves but as a whole complex or biosystem. When the biosystem is fragmented, the organism dies. Each component of a biosystem helps create the context and the frequency of the biosystem. Whole herbs possess this "aura," whereas the active element alone of a herb only contributes a portion of the whole.

This is why the effects of some herbs are listed as unknown or may be varied. For example, dandelion (*Taraxacum officinale*) is traditionally used as a diuretic to increase urinary volume, and as a choleretic to stimulate bile production and facilitate the digestion of fats. These two effects stem from three active ingredients. These are lactucopicrin, a natural diuretic; taraxacin, which increases urinary volume; and a natural bitter that stimulates bile production. What the active principle relieves can be seen, but what the whole herb may accomplish does not always coincide with the listed actions of the active principles of that herb. For instance, dandelion is listed for treating cellulitis, high cholesterol, constipation, liver ailments, gout, hemorrhoids, certain skin conditions, rheumatism, and obesity. Its constituents include chlorophyll, an alkaloid, an essential oil, beta carotene, vitamins B and C, inulin, minerals, tannin, and glycosides. The synergy of these components and the energy pattern of the whole plant contribute to the therapeutic value of dandelion, which may be used successfully for any one of the listed ailments. *With whole herbs, the natural and entire medicinal value of the plant is retained, whereas a single allopathic drug provides only partial and imbalanced therapy.*

This "whole medicinal value" of a plant is very important, for in nature, there are some dangerous or poisonous substances. Many plants used therapeutically contain poisonous substances as part of their complex, but the interaction of their components enhances the effects of helpful substances while reducing those of harmful ones. A report by the American Council on Science and Health has revealed countless examples of carcinogens and mutagens found in nature. According to the council's definition, a carcinogen is considered to be "any substance that significantly increases the incidence of any type of tumor in any one animal species at any dose level." A mutagen is a substance that produces damage to the genetic material known as DNA, causing cell death or causing the cell to become a cancerous cell. A mutational test (the Ames test) involves the inoculation of the questionable substance into a strain of bacterium called *Salmonella typhimurium*.

Be aware that testing, especially for government regulation, involves the investigation of the worst possible case, which usually means feeding the substance in question at *abnormally high doses*. A substance will be considered carcinogenic if a significant increase in tumors occurs, even if the animal dies of old age. Moreover, *the regulatory decision will not be reversed even if evidence in humans negates animal findings*. If an animal test reveals even a single case of tumors from a substance under investigation, it will be branded a hazard and a carcinogen.

The problem with this mode of investigation is that it uses isolated compounds that do not include the whole value of the biosystem and the influences from the integration of all components. In addition, researchers rarely consider "normal" exposure or consumption of these products. Tests can also be conducted by administering the substance under investigation through drinking water, inhalation, injection, skin painting, or some other route. *Many of the substances considered carcinogenic or mutagenic by governments are considered therapeutic by biotechnological laboratories*. One flagrant example is quercitin. Quercetin is a bioflavonoid—a chemical compound found in many plants. In the council's report, quercetin is listed as being highly mutagenic. On the flip side, a study published in the *Journal of Immunology* in 1981 found quercetin to be the most potent bioflavonoid tested in reducing the production of histamine, which suppresses allergic reactions. Another study, published in *Biochemical Pharmacology* in 1983, declared that quercetin was an antioxidant, preventing harmful chemical reactions that can damage cells and tissues. All three of these studies are of equal scientific integrity, but they bear conflicting results.

This is a good example of the differences between allopathic and holistic methods and medicine. Holistic medicine treats the context of the cells and considers the entire system of treatment, incorporating all elements and components of the context. Allopathic medicine bases its findings on double-blind tests that carry out investigations in a controlled environment (which is not the animal's natural environment), considering only a single element or predetermined factors. But as the feeding of a substance in macrodoses is an unlikely situation in nature, how relevant are the results? *Overconsumption of any product, even those evaluated as being good for you, is likely to cause illness.* When elements are taken in the proper balance, they are more likely to do some good. The principle of holistic investigation is in fact to maintain the most natural balance for the particular species in its natural environment.

Moreover, mutagenicity implies the production of free radical reactions, which damage DNA. Although it is known that antioxidants, such as quercetin and vitamin C, cause free radical reactions in the test tube, in the organism itself, anti-oxidants block free radical reactions and defuse free-floating free radicals. This is an excellent demonstration of the subtle mechanisms associated with "whole" biosystems and their natural environments.

Dosage plays a critical role in the safety of these controversial substances. Unfortunately, few studies of dosages have been performed in either humans or animals. Dosages must be more thoroughly investigated in both holistic and allopathic studies. Factors that influence dosage include lifestyle, diet, disease state, stress, and environment.

STANDARDIZED HERBS

The types and amounts of active principles a herb contains depend on soil condition, climate, the plant parts used, harvesting methods, pro-

cessing, and packaging. Because of these factors, it is essential for manufacturers to have a control system. Of course manufacturers who grow their own stock can control the quality of the main ingredients of their remedies. Other responsible companies batch-test for residues, consistency, and purity. But especially when one is dealing with active constituents in herbal preparations, it is necessary to have some sort of standardization. Because certain ingredients in herbs may be dangerous if consumed in high concentrations, the establishment of safe concentrations is necessary. This had led to the introduction of standardized herbs.

The active principles of standardized herbs are identified with such tests as chromatographic analysis. This type of batch-testing is done by the manufacturer's laboratory or through an independent laboratory. Concentrations of active principles are listed on the product labels only by those manufacturers that adhere to standardization. Manufacturers are not obligated to test herbs for active principles; those manufacturers that do conduct such tests do so voluntarily.

PYRAMID OF HERBS

The diagram includes some plants commonly used as teas. To explain the therapeutic uses of each herb would itself require an entire volume. This pyramid condenses some of the information and identifies the part of the body in which the herb is known to be most effective.

Many books on herbs reveal the pharmacological nature of the herb and whether it is antispasmodic, decongestive, and so on. Each herb also has a specific direction and usually affects a certain area of the body more readily than another. This natural direction is preserved in dried whole herbs.

Brain/Nervous System

Eucalyptus, peppermint, skullcap, yarrow, lunden, rosehip.

Heart/Cardio-vascular System

Comfrey, hawthorn, ginseng.

Broncho-pulmonary System

Eucalyptus, rosemary, couch grass, scabwort, horse chestnut.

Liver/Gallbladder

Dandelion, artichoke, angelica, golden seal, peppermint.

Stomach

Angelica, chamomile, ginseng, licorice, peppermint.

Intestine

Golden seal, licorice, yarrow, mallow, wallwort, strawberry leaves, raspberry leaves.

Urogenital System

Golden seal, ginseng, chamomile.

FOR FURTHER READING

Pryor, W., ed. *Free Radicals in Biology, vol.* VI. Orlando, Fla.: Academic Press, 1984.

Shin, H. W., et al. "Studies on Inorganic Composition and Immunopotentiating Activity of *Ganoderma lucidum* in Korea." *Korean Journal of Pharmacology* 14 (1985).

Wagner, H.; Zenk, M. H.; and Ott, H. "Polysaccharides Derived from *Echinacea* Plants As Immunostimulants." *Patent-Ger Often* 3 (1988).

Weiner, M. *Earth medicine.* New York: Macmillan, 1972.

Weiner, M. *Weiner's Herbal Nutrition against Aging.* Boston: Houghton-Mifflin, 1986.

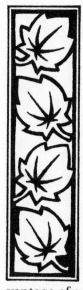

EIGHT

Tinctures
and Extracts

Tinctures carry the therapeutic properties of the plants that they are made from. The advantage of a tincture is that it is in liquid form and is absorbed by the bloodstream faster than the solid herb. Moreover, a tincture can be made up of several plants, yielding a specific combination of therapeutic properties.

Tinctures are alcohol percolations of fresh plants that yield remedies. Chapter 1 explains the basic preparation of a tincture, which consists of soaking plant parts in a solvent such as alcohol to separate the active principles of the plant. The concentration of alcohol contained in a tincture depends on the chemical nature of the active principles in the plants. These active principles have a solubility factor that determines at what concentration of alcohol they will dissolve in solution.

Most tinctures contain 50 percent alcohol. Research by certain manufacturers has shown that tinctures with a concentration of alcohol less than 50 percent are subject to microbial activity. Bacteria alter substances, often causing fermentation of sugars. If this occurred, the extract would be contaminated, or at least have altered properties. Thus, a generous content of alcohol is necessary for product longevity. Tinctures are taken by the *drop,* and thus the alcohol consumption with such remedies is not high. Nevertheless, because of their alcohol content, tinctures are not prescribed for alcoholics and are not recommended for infants, who might become habituated to them.

Tinctures require extra care in their preparation, as well as chromatographic and other chemical testing to ensure the quality of their active ingredients. Only reputable manufacturers, mostly established Swiss companies, follow these "checking" procedures. *It is important to look for manufacturing claims on tinctures, since alcohol alters certain of the active principles contained in plants.* For instance, if the alcohol extraction of echinacea is not properly prepared, the polysaccharide that stimulates the production of interferon and T-cell lymphocytes will be precipitated out of solution. Likewise, certain plant pigments are altered or discolored through alcohol extraction.

Quality control is of the utmost importance in the manufacturing of tinctures. Fresh plants are the raw materials and main ingredients of tinctures, and we know that the chemical makeup of plants depends on their geographical location, the weather, the period of harvest, the conditions of soil, the plant's life stage, and the part of the plant used. For a consistent product, manufacturers of tinctures must control their raw materials. Plants used in tinctures should be organically grown, and if wild varieties are used, soil samples must be checked for toxic residues and the resultant tinctures batch-tested for such residues. Pollutants, chemicals, and radioactive substances are dangerous to one's health and undermine the value of the remedy.

Tinctures are very active substances because they usually use fresh plants and thus carry all the imprints and energy of the original biosystem. Furthermore, no drying or processes involving heat or light, which may destroy or alter the energy imprint and the active components of the plants, are used.

LIXIVIATION FOR NONSOLVENT EXTRACTS

Most tinctures and extracts are produced by placing macerated plants in a solvent—alcohol or ether—and allowing the active principles to separate out. *Tinctures usually use fresh plants, whereas extracts use dried plant parts that are first powdered and then soaked in alcohol.*

A true extract is made through lixiviation. In this process, plant parts are separated and dried. Usually herbs are air-dried, but today's technology allows them to be freeze-dried. Steam is then forced through the powdered, dried plant, and the solution collected is the extract. The extract produced is sometimes further reduced by boiling to the desired concentration.

Lixiviation produces alcohol-free extracts, but the process involves high temperatures that destroy many active ingredients such as flavonoids and volatile oils. This process is usually used for prescription remedies prepared by herbalists or chemists for the inclusion in a herbal complex. Pure, undiluted extracts are rarely available commercially; these are too concentrated and difficult for the layperson to dose. Furthermore, they must be analyzed chromatographically to determine the exact content of active ingredients.

THE BIOLOGICAL PATHWAYS OF TINCTURES AND EXTRACTS

Here tinctures and extracts are discussed interchangeably, for biologically they react the same way. Tinctures are classified as reacting at the organ level. But unlike allopathic drugs, they adapt to the body. All activity in the biosystem begins at the cellular level, but some remedies also have an influence at the tissue level of specific organs.

Although you receive a "whole environment" when you take freeze-dried herbs, because they are in capsule form they often will contain excipients, which must be eliminated and therefore use energy. *Tinctures are in liquid form, with an almost immediate action on the body, because they require little digestion.* The active ingredients from a tincture will enter the bloodstream three to five times faster than the same ingredients in solid form.

Tinctures resemble allopathic drugs in that the levels of their doses are shown in the blood. Unlike homeopathic remedies, tinctures are undiluted—they are the mother tincture. The higher the dose of tincture or extract, the higher the blood level of active ingredients.

Because tinctures use the whole plant, they contain its original balance of chemicals, providing a system that counteracts those active ingredients that are dangerous.

Tinctures are used for chronic as well as periodic illnesses. Because of their high medicinal value, tinctures are good remedies for relieving symptoms. But unlike allopathic drugs, tinctures also help the body heal while relieving symptoms.

Most tinctures are made of a combination of plants, known as a herbal complex, giving tinctures the advantages of synergy. Combinations of different plants within one remedy also provide adjuvant therapy, a major factor in the pharmacodynamics of tinctures. Adjuvant therapy allows the main ingredient in the tincture to be reinforced by one or more plants, which will either enhance the effectiveness of the main ingredient or give supportive treatment to the secondary symptoms of a particular illness. For example, let's say a herbal preparation for cardiac weakness is needed. A weak heart may be due to age, convalescence from disease, stress, diet, or exercise. Most natural-remedy amateurs would quickly name hawthorn *(Crataegus oxyacantha)* as the main ingredient for a cardiac remedy. *For centuries, hawthorn has been recommended for cardiac problems, mainly because it contains flavonoids that enlarge the coronary vessels.* If the coronary vessels are enlarged, the blood flows to the heart more easily, and consequently more oxygen will be carried to the heart. If the heart gets more oxygen, coronary stress is relieved. This also relieves physical symptoms of anxiety which are almost always present during cardiac insufficiency. But what about the swelling with edema that might occur because of cardiac insufficiency? Hawthorn does nothing for swelling. A plant that contains a nitritelike substance to re-establish the metabolism of the heart would add to the efficacy of the remedy. So we could add cactus or holly or both of these plants as adjuvants to our main ingredient—hawthorn. But cardiac insufficiency also makes the patient anxious. Anxiety can affect the nervous system and provoke overstimulation, jangled nerves, uncontrolled reflexes, and excitability. A plant that would calm the system would in effect prepare the system for treatment with the main ingredient. So we could add some oat *(Avena sativa)* extract or some valerian. And for a well-rounded herbal complex, we would include a cardiac tonic, such as camphor. With this mixture, all the bases are covered, and we can describe the herbal complex as a holistic remedy.

Another example of the holistic nature of tinctures is a remedy for constipation. For chronic constipation, it is most important to find the reason for the problem. Nevertheless, any remedy for constipation, whether chronic or occasional, must not shock the system into elimination and must not be habit forming. It must redirect the body systems involved.

A laxative particularly needs adjuvant ingredients to cope with the secondary reactions of constipation, which may include liver congestion due to toxicity from substances that have not been eliminated; inflammation of the mucosa; poor appetite; decreased movement (peristalsis) of the intestine; and vitamin deficiencies. Senna is ideal as the main ingredient, because it contains a glycoside, causing peristaltic movement that becomes active under the influence of the intestinal bacteria. It is active only in the large intestine and does not burn or alter the biochemical nature of any other part of the digestive tract. A laxative should also contain a stool softener. Many plant substances containing mucilage-type fiber could be used. Buckthorn *(Rhamnus cathartica)* is useful because it also stimulates the gallbladder and therefore is an adjuvant, providing relief of liver congestion. Dandelion and bearberry (*Arctostaphylos uva-ursi*) could also be included as supportive treatment. Pressure on the urinary system often occurs from constipation. Dandelion increases urine volume by 40 percent, thereby clearing the system and preventing painful pressure while it promotes liver function. Bearberry destroys bacteria specific to the bladder and promotes kidney function.

These examples show how tinctures provide relief of symptoms by healing the system, which is the ultimate goal of a holistic remedy.

The form of each remedy provides advantages and disadvantages. Tinctures are devoid of some of the plant substances contained within the original fresh plant because these substances are destroyed by alcohol or they are altered by continued enzymatic activity. At the same time, the liquid form of a tincture is the fastest means for the body to absorb plant substances because in contrast to solid herbal remedies, little digestion is required for these materials to reach the bloodstream.

FOR FURTHER READING

Morrison, R. T., and Boyd, R. N. *Organic Chemistry.* Boston: Allyn and Bacon, 1973.

NINE

Vitamins, Minerals, and Nutrients

VITAMINS

Vitamins are essential to the proper growth and maintenance of our bodies. With a few exceptions, vitamins cannot be synthesized by the human body, but must be supplied from a balanced diet or from supplements. When the body synthesizes a particular substance, it uses raw materials supplied by the foods we eat to create that substance. With vitamins, however, the body must use already-formed vitamin molecules that are provided by the breakdown of food or by vitamin supplements. The body uses these molecules whole; it does not assemble molecules to make the vitamin.

Vitamins are important in many biochemical reactions essential to body functioning. They may be needed for optimum enzyme activity, which catalyzes biochemical reactions. For a cell to function properly, it must be properly nourished. Enzyme deficiencies can lead to cell malfunction, which, if very prolonged or severe, can ultimately lead to cell death. This explains why the symptoms of vitamin deficiencies appear over an extended period of time. Likewise, *ailments or diseases linked to cellular malfunctioning due to a lack of coenzyme-vitamin occur over a period of many years.* The decline and death of one cell leads to the death of other cells and to the deterioration of tissues and organs, and consequently of the entire biosystem.

Many vitamins contain a metallic ion that allows them to transfer electrons. This transfer of electrons traps energy from the breakdown of foods in the form of energy-rich chemical compounds that the body uses for various functions. This aids in changing the energy pattern of the body so that the body can resonate at its optimally healthful frequency. Biochemical reactions involving electron transfer are also essential to cellular respiration—the breath of life of the biosystem. That these biochemical processes depend on vitamins demonstrate how vitamins are essential to us.

This interrelation of processes within the human body involving vitamins brings up the controversy of whether it is necessary to supplement vitamins. On one side of the controversy, the traditionalists believe that it is possible to obtain all necessary vitamins from a well-rounded diet—a diet composed of the four basic food groups. Those on the other side believe in all kinds of vitamin and food supplements, often in megadoses, nursing the distinct impression that these supplements will multiply the individual's energy, endurance, and muscle mass. We know that it is impossible to get even basic amounts of many vitamins from the foods we eat. For instance, it would be necessary to eat one pound of wheat germ to get 50 milligrams of vitamin E, and in this fast-paced age it is practically impossible to always get an adequate diet. Moreover, food costs prevent the consumption of many foods that are better sources of certain vitamins. Soils polluted by pesticides and herbicides further lower the quality of our foods, destroying many vitamins. Refrigeration, processing, and simple cooking of many fresh foods also destroys vitamins. It is clear that eating the right food alone is not the optimum method of securing the necessary vitamins.

Of course indiscriminately consuming any vitamin supplement on the market is not the answer either, because there are significant differences between vitamin products. There are also dangers with liberal dosing of vitamins. As with all remedies, an adequate balance is essential. This balance is perhaps more important with vitamins than with any other natural product, and it is certainly more intricate.

Fat Soluble or Water Soluble?

Vitamins are either fat soluble or water soluble. Water-soluble vitamins dissolve in water. They are much easier to assimilate, since they dissolve in the digestive tract and for the most part are absorbed immediately by the bloodstream. In contrast, fat-soluble vitamins must be carried on a lipid (fat) molecule to be assimilated. The digestive process is long, and fat-soluble vitamins must bind with bile salts and fats to be absorbed.

With water-soluble vitamins, quantities are measured in milligrams. The units of measurement for fat-soluble vitamins are international units (IU). So *when a label gives the concentration of a vitamin in milligrams, you know it is a water-soluble vitamin.* Beta carotene is the exception; it is a water-soluble vitamin measured in international units, because it is a derivative of fat-soluble vitamin A.

Recommended Dietary Allowances (RDAs)

Recommended Dietary Allowances (RDAs) are the minimum amounts of vitamins or minerals that are thought to prevent deficiencies of those vitamins or minerals. These minimum values have been set through the study of vitamin deficiency. The standards for RDAs are set by the Food and Nutrition Board of the National Research Council in the United States and by Health and Welfare Canada. The action, benefits, and possible therapeutic value of the vitamin were not considered in these studies.

This narrow view of vitamin therapy is a weak standard. Preventing vitamin deficiency is not an approach that will bring about an optimum resonance of the body; it will merely maintain it in a neutral state. For the most part, the RDA values can be filled by consuming a "balanced diet" that incorporates the basic food groups.

Few vitamins are toxic, and overconsumption of most will result in their excretion via urine. Some vitamins are stored in the body, where they remain until they can be used. Yet others, notably vitamin A and vitamin D, can be toxic or cause detriment to the biosystem if taken in excess. For example, overconsumption of vitamin D can cause calcification of soft tissues in the heart and lungs and calcification of the walls of blood vessels and kidney tubules, leading to pathological changes in these organs. However, *vitamins A and D are the only "dangerous" vitamins, and amounts as high as five times RDA values, over long periods of time, have been deemed safe.* Symptoms associated with overdose of vitamins, such as the headache, dry skin, and fatigue seen in vitamin A toxicity, for instance, will disappear within a few days, once overconsumption has been terminated.

Be aware that toxic doses of vitamins far exceed the RDA amounts, and large amounts must be consumed over several months before symptoms of toxicity become apparent.

Although excess vitamins are eliminated, consuming too many vitamins and minerals may pose a problem. According to the theory of entropy, too many biochemical reactions lead to chaos in the biosystem. When there are too many vitamins, there is a surplus of coenzymes. These coenzymes must bond with a protein, causing a biochemical reaction. In addition, eliminating excess vitamins requires energy. This increase in biochemical reactions, along with the energy used in the reactions and the elimination of excess vitamins, leads to entropy and the counteracting of the vitamins' benefits. This is not to say that vitamin supplementation is bad, or that therapeutically prescribed megadoses of vitamins are noneffective. It only suggests that liberal use of megadoses may lead to entropy, canceling the nutritional benefits of vitamins.

The Difference between Holistic and Allopathic Use of Vitamins

Allopathic medicine uses vitamins to treat vitamin deficiencies. Holistic medicine uses vitamins therapeutically, for the prevention of disease, and to increase resistance to biosocial and ecological factors such as pollution and stress. Whereas allopathic physicians prescribe RDA levels of vitamins to maintain cellular functioning and the neutral (not optimal) state of the organism, holistic physicians use megadoses of certain vitamins as therapeutic agents in the treatment of certain diseases. For example, much emphasis and scientific investigation has been placed on the cardiovascular benefits of fish oils. Many scientific studies on humans indicate that fish oils are useful in the prevention and treatment of heart disease, stroke, and high blood pressure. Scientific investigation was driven by the observation that Eskimo and Japanese populations have a very low incidence of heart disease, and this was attributed to their high intake of fish. One study by Sanders, published in *Clinical Science* in 1983, at the height of the fish oil craze, revealed that fish oils changed the blood-lipid profile. The blood-lipid profile refers to fat content of the blood. *Since fish oils improve the cholesterol ratio of the blood, the heart is not taxed.* Moreover, fish oils reduce clotting, the main cause of stroke. Many other scientifically documented cases of treatment with vitamin therapy have won the attention of staunch allopathic practitioners, causing the therapeutic achievements of vitamin therapy to spill over to allopathic medicine.

Many physicians recognize the data resulting from the scientific investigation of vitamins. In a sense, vitamins are like herbs. But although they have many therapeutic and pharmacologic effects, they have the advantage of being manufactured and endorsed by pharmaceutical companies. A mighty pharmaceutical entity can spend millions of dollars researching a drug or a vitamin, and the dissemination of data from these sources is well respected, especially by governments. For this reason, more allopathic doctors believe in vitamin and mineral therapy than in herb therapy. Vitamins work along allopathic lines, and they may be used as drugs.

The introduction into your diet of one vitamin may cause your body to call for the increase of another vitamin. High vitamin levels may have a therapeutic effect on the body, whereas low doses may not affect physiological responses at all. The manipulation of molecules in the body that occurs during vitamin therapy is so akin to what occurs with allopathic medicine that it has caused governments to make recommendations for the use of vitamins and minerals, in the form of RDAs. Indeed, there are volumes of current research on the therapeutics of certain vitamins and minerals, but most of the time, this therapeutic effect of a vitamin is achieved with doses that can be 50 to 100 times greater than the prescribed RDA value. At these levels, vitamins and minerals can be dangerous. Like drugs, they can have certain contraindications. They can be helpful for one condition but have detrimental effects for other body mechanisms. In a sense, government restrictions help to provide insurance that only qualified specialists will prescribe megadoses. Qualified specialists may not necessarily be allopathic physicians, but they must understand nutrition and physiology and be aware of all the research data on vitamin therapy.

MINERALS

Minerals help to make up our bones, teeth, soft tissue, muscle, blood, and nerve cells. They are important for physiological processes and may even be considered the spark plugs in biochemical reactions. Minerals monitor the passage of substances in and out of cells. They are particularly important in maintaining water balance. There are 17 minerals that are essential to the proper functioning of mental and physical processes in the human body, and they must be supplied in the diet.

Minerals are always measured in milligrams and micrograms. Some minerals are found as parts of vitamins. For example, vitamin B_1 contains the mineral sulfur. *All minerals are interrelated, and no one mineral can act without affecting another mineral in the body.* For example, copper helps iron to transport oxygen via hemoglobin. Also, copper and calcium must be present for iron to function. Furthermore, vitamins interact with minerals. For instance, vitamin C helps the absorption of iron, and copper metabolizes vitamin C into forming elastin, a protein that is the chief constituent of connective tissue. Manganese metabolizes biotin, thiamine, and vitamin C. It is therefore impossible to consider vitamins and minerals as separate entities.

Some minerals are referred to as trace minerals because they are present in the body in minute amounts and even therapeutically are required only in minute amounts. Trace minerals are measured in micrograms.

The balance between the interaction of minerals and that of minerals and vitamins is so delicate that liberal dosing or self-treatment with vitamins and minerals should never be attempted without professional advice. Not only do vitamins and minerals interact with each other, but they are also affected by drugs, foods that you ingest, and pollutants that you're exposed to. For instance, fiber in foods, antacids, and the industrial pollutants cadmium and lead are known to be iron inhibitors.

The foods you eat and the beverages you drink can sometimes interfere with absorption of capsules, and this depends on the contents of the capsule, not on the gelatin capsule. For example, a zinc supplement taken with an iron supplement will bind to the iron and carry it out of the body, thus reducing the intake of zinc and using up the iron as well as some of your body's energy. The same thinking advises against taking ginseng capsules after eating vegetables or fruits, or before drinking citrus juices. The vitamin C in these foods will deplete the ginseng, and cancel the benefits of the supplement. You can avoid this interaction between substances by taking supplements at different times during the day, or by taking time-released capsules.

Often several interrelating ingredients are combined in a capsule using a medical time-release gel to coat each of the elements, because the gel causes the ingredient to dissolve only when a calculated amount of time has elapsed after you swallow the capsule. You can recognize such capsules because they contain small beads of different colors. The colored beads are different elements or active ingredients, color coated to dissolve and to be released at specific times after ingestion.

A table at the end of this chapter shows the nature of the vitamin-mineral interactions. Keep in mind that for beneficial and therapeutic effects to take place, not only must the interacting substance be present, but it must be present at the adequate level. Even a minor change in concentration can produce an upset in the delicate biochemical balance. Furthermore, *when too much of a vitamin or another interacting substance is absorbed, it will throw off the biochemical balance of other substances, setting off a chain reaction and leading to complete havoc of biochemical processes.*

ESTABLISHING A NUTRIENT PROFILE

It is important to remember that all nutrients—vitamins, minerals, trace elements, and amino acids—interrelate within our biosystem. To get a clear picture of anyone's nutritional status, each nutrient must be viewed as it relates to another. This is a complex procedure requiring medical differential diagnosis—for example, by testing blood sugar levels after single-food "meals," to find out what internal reactions occur under the influence of certain nutrients. Or by testing blood pressure after exposure to pollutants, together with a patient's report of associated sensations, such as dizziness or fluctuating emotions. Or by urine analysis for amino acid content, and a hair-sample biopsy for mineral content. Without this type of medical differential diagnostic testing, often referred to as ecologic-metabolic workup, an exact nutrient profile cannot be accomplished, and the prescription of supplements for therapeutic purposes will be mere guesswork. Today there are more physicians practicing medical differential diagnosis than in the past. They are medical doctors who subscribe to holistic and nutritional therapy. You could inquire at the Holistic Medical Association closest to your area or at an association of ecological medical practitioners for the names of registered practitioners.

NATURAL OR SYNTHETIC SUPPLEMENTS?

As with all other natural remedies, the process by which vitamins and minerals are manufactured plays an important role in the efficacy of a product. The quality of raw materials used in the manufacture of vitamins and minerals is equally important. Vitamin and mineral supplementation became fashionable in the 1980s, leading health food and pharmaceutical companies to flood the market with "exciting, revolutionary" supplements. Most of the new products were simply carbon copies or poor reproductions of long-existing vitamins and minerals. The craze prompted investigation by major government and university research institutes, who studied the effects of vitamins and minerals on the body and looked closely at their therapeutic possibilities. Many new facts were discovered that have led to the evolution of nutrient supplementation which is now in full swing.

Benefits of Synthetic Supplements

There are basically two types of supplements: pharmaceutical and organic. Several patented processes exclusive to each manufacturer exist within each category. Essentially, pharmaceutical vitamins and minerals are synthetically produced, and their active ingredient is produced in the laboratory. The highest-quality synthetic form of vitamin is designated on labels as "pure crystalline." This means that under an electron microscope, the vitamin or mineral powder appears as crystals. *Synthetic vitamins and minerals are not necessarily bad. In fact, they are advantageous for people suffering from food allergies and intolerances,* for they contain no nutrients that may be troublesome to the allergic individual. Virtually all B and C vitamins are synthetically produced. As you now know, producing some vitamins from food sources requires huge amounts of foods—for example, four pounds of rice to obtain only 50 milligrams of a B vitamin. Considering the number of vitamin manufacturers and the high dosages of vitamins available on the market today, using food sources would deplete the world food supply within a very short time.

Benefits of Semisynthetic Vitamins

Other vitamins are semisynthetic, meaning that they are produced in a laboratory but that nutrient-extracted vitamins or minerals are added. Vitamin C (ascorbic acid) is the best example of this type of vitamin. Virtually all vitamin C is produced in the laboratory, but many companies claim that their vitamin C is from natural sources. In fact, it is a synthetically produced ascorbic acid combined with a small amount of vitamin C extracted from fruit or herbs, or more commonly, whole fruit or herbs, such as acerola or rose hips, are added. This small added proportion of natural vitamin C serves two purposes: it helps the body assimilate the synthetic ascorbic acid, and it provides the body with the energy pattern of the biosystem it was extracted from, thus contributing vital energy frequencies.

Organic Vitamins and Minerals

Organic vitamins and minerals are nutrients that have been isolated from organic substances found in nature, having been extracted from plant and animal tissues. Either such substances may have been produced under organic growth conditions, or they were mass-cultivated. The same problem that was discussed earlier also exists when comparing organic and mass-cultivated foods. A lack of control over soil, water, and growth conditions may make plants toxic. Dangerous toxins from polluted areas may infiltrate the plants and then be stored by the plants. However, it is difficult to learn whether a vitamin or mineral has been manufactured with organic substances, and the only proof is the manufacturer's word on the label. Manufacturers of "natural" or organic vitamins proclaim their organic growth measures, or claim that batches have been bio-assayed for chemical residues. They will state this on labels or in brochures. (If a company claims to use organic ingredients with no harmful residues, it knows that its competitors will buy the product and send it for analysis.)

When you consider the toxic residues in the raw materials used to manufacture vitamins, you realize that *pharmaceutical-grade vitamins may have an advantage over the organic nutrients, since they are pure crystalline chemicals, uncontaminated by pollutants.*

Benefits of Organic Vitamins and Minerals

However, the energy and assimilation levels of "natural" and synthetic vitamins are very different. Substances extracted from natural biosystems will contribute their energy pattern to the body, whereas synthetically derived ones do not. Although natural source vitamins may contribute allergens to sensitive individuals, for most people they create fewer gastrointestinal upsets and fewer toxic reactions than do synthetic vitamins, especially when they must be taken in large doses for therapeutic treatment. We cannot liken synthetic vitamins to drugs, because they do not have a biphasic effect. They provide nutrients, as do foods, rather than foreign molecules, as do "drug" substances unknown to our bodies. Synthetic vitamins can cause toxicity as drugs can, unlike their natural counterpart. Aspirin has been shown to cause acidity and toxicity of the stomach, whereas its naturally occurring counterpart, salicin (from willow bark), is only changed into salicylic acid in the intestine, thus bypassing the stomach and averting stomach acidity. Similarly, some studies have shown that natural vitamin E is absorbed by the body from 12 to 20 times more effectively than synthetic E. However, people who are allergic or intolerant to soya will get a negative reaction from natural vitamin E, which is derived from soya.

Herbs As Vitamin and Mineral Sources

Today manufacturers often use herbs as sources of vitamins and minerals. This is a natural option, since *for over 2,000 years the Chinese have considered herbs and plants as healing foods*. Supplements are now coming out with herbal formulae that combine a number of different herbs. The important thing to look for when you are choosing formulas is a standardization guarantee on labels. Standardization simply means that the whole herb has been used, as opposed to the active principle only. As discussed earlier, extraction changes the energy pattern of the substance, reducing the benefits associated with the other principles contained in the plant. By using the entire herb, the formula is better assimilated by the body, because of the complementary energy pattern and natural balance or synergy contained in the herb. This standardization is usually expressed on a label as "certified potency." It guarantees that quality is consistent and that the herbs have been grown under controlled conditions, as well as ensuring their full potency by use of the whole herb.

Chlorella and Other Valuable Nutrients

Other forms of supplements come in a sort of miscellaneous category commonly called nutrients. These are the multivitamin complexes made from dehydrated or specially processed whole foods, such as algae, mushrooms, or yeast. They contain many vitamins and minerals, as well as other constituents. One of the best examples is chlorella, a microalgae with an impressive nutritional profile. Chlorella contains vitamins B_1, B_2, B_3, B_5 (pantothenic acid), B_6, C, E, folic acid, biotin, PABA, and inositol. A typical 100-gram sample of chlorella contains 125 micrograms of vitamin B_{12} and 55,000 IU of vitamin A, and 221 milligrams of calcium, 315 milligrams of magnesium, 30 milligrams of iron, 71 milligrams of zinc, 0.4 milligrams of iodine, and 895 milligrams of phosphorus. It is also a rich source of amino acids. Chlorella has been used therapeutically with remarkable success in treating such ailments as arthritis, memory loss, depression, vision problems, heart problems, and emphysema. This single-celled freshwater algae was found to reverse and even cure some people afflicted with degenerative diseases such as arthritis and deteriorating vision. Researchers believe that chlorella's beneficial effect lies in its content of nucleic acids.

DNA and RNA

Nucleic acids, otherwise known as DNA (deoxyribonucleic acid) and RNA (ribonucleic acid), have the same structure in all living systems. The breakdown of these acids in our bodies provides us with the building blocks essential to health. Moreover, they do so in a balanced way, without the guesswork of molecular manipulation, because structurally, the breakdown of RNA and DNA is identical for all biosystems. They provide the constituents necessary for the repair and replacement of the cellular nucleic acids that are essential to our cells' functioning. The energy pattern found in chlorella is highly compatible with most living organisms, because of the presence of high concentrations of RNA and DNA. Chlorella contains about 10 percent RNA and 3 percent DNA.

Chlorella's Many Benefits

From this nutrient profile, we can clearly see how chlorella can be marketed as a supplement. It is, in fact, more than a multivitamin complex. Chlorella is also considered to be an antioxidant because of its high content of chlorophyll—a known detoxifying agent. Because it is such an effective detoxifying agent, it has been used in Taiwan to decontaminate well water. It follows that *chlorella provides protection against environmental pollutants found in food, in water, and in the air.* Chlorella is also used as a growth factor. It is a natural source of the "chlorella growth factor," isolated in 1950 at the People's Scientific Research Center in Tokyo. Small animals fed a 10 percent solution of chlorella showed a 10 percent to 47 percent increase in growth.

Other Nutrients

There are many nutrient substances like chlorella that are marketed as supplements, which are not categorized as either whole foods or herbs. They include choline or lecithin, chlorophyll, and yeast. Many such nutrients are marketed as "workout" products aimed at athletes and body builders. These may include gamma-oryzanol—a white powder extracted from rice-bran oil, used as an antioxidant by serious athletes, and glucose polymer—a complex carbohydrate derived from corn, used instead of sugared drinks to enhance water and carbohydrate absorption during workouts.

Vitamin Sources and Combinations

Unfortunately, among natural remedies, the labeling of vitamins and minerals can be the most ambiguous. *Vitamins claiming to be from natural sources are usually synthetic, with additions of natural sources.* All forms of vitamin C and any of the B vitamins are synthetically produced; some are simply supplemented with natural source nutrients. Vitamins that are really derived from natural sources are sometimes called "megafoods," or "whole-food vitamins," and the label clearly explains that they have been derived from certain food sources—for example, calcium from oyster shells. Other labels describe vitamins in chemical terms, and in such cases, it is essential to know something about chemistry. The most common example of this is vitamin E, which is known as tocopherol. Synthetic vitamin E is DL-alpha tocopherol, whereas naturally derived vitamin E is D-alpha tocopherol. The omission of the "L" in the derived vitamin indicates a major difference in the origin of this vitamin and in its assimilation and action in the body.

Still other vitamins have special "synergistic" combinations. Synergy is the enhancement of one ingredient by the presence of another. Such combinations may be synthetically or naturally derived, and what is important is their combinations. They are teamed up with enzymes to help speed up biochemical reactions and in some cases help the digestion of a fat-soluble vitamin, or an additional nutrient or herb. Other combinations include vitamins and the minerals necessary for their assimilation. Still others include minerals that act to buffer the vitamin. For instance, *vitamin C may be buffered with calcium, magnesium, and potassium, because these buffering minerals reduce the acidity of the ascorbic acid and prevent corrosion of the teeth.*

Antiallergy Vitamins

Today's vitamins and minerals can be classed as either regular or antiallergy vitamins. Antiallergy vitamins are derived synthetically and are developed with food allergies and intolerance in mind. It is now known that food allergies and intolerances are physiological, not psychosomatic, ailments, and it is important to understand the allergy mechanism.

An estimated 40 million North Americans suffer from food allergies. Recent research reveals that two out of three individuals are sensitive to some chemical found in common nutrients. It has been shown that coumarin, a substance found in wheat, cheese, beef, eggs, and food dyes causes digestive disturbances and distress, notably bloating. This is an example of what is known as food intolerance, in which a substance found in foods, even though it may be a commonly used nutrient will cause a negative physiological reaction. Food intolerances are generally not life threatening, but they cause enough distress to warrant avoidance of the substance.

An allergy, in contrast, can be life threatening. An allergen is a substance that causes an allergic reaction. Exposure to the allergen initiates the production of the immunoglobulin IgE, which causes the mast cells to release chemicals called mediators—leukotrienes and histamine. These mediators cause specific biological reactions, which we recognize as the symptoms associated with allergies.

Leukotrienes cause the lungs to construct, resulting in difficult breathing, congestion of the chest cavity, coughing, and wheezing.

Histamine produces edema (swelling) by causing the capillary walls to become flaccid and allowing liquid to pass through and accumulate in the surrounding tissue. This results in swelling of mucous membranes of the nose and the eyes, and weals on the skin. This leaking of fluid from blood vessels lowers the blood pressure, causing fatigue, and possibly, if pressure descends too low, anaphylactic shock. Histamine also causes constriction of the smooth muscles of the lungs, resulting in spasms that manifest as coughing, choking, and difficult breathing. Histamine also causes the release of hydrochloric acid, which results in the diarrhea and intestinal cramps often associated with allergies.

Vitamin Therapy for Allergy

There are many supplements that can help to prevent allergic reactions. For example, bioflavonoids have been proven to inhibit the release of histamine, to prevent histamine-induced permeability of capillaries, and to inhibit anaphylaxis. *Vitamin therapy to treat allergic individuals is very common today and is becoming an important branch of medicine and nutritional healing.* Because vitamin C suppresses the release of corticoid hormones, it assists in the proper functioning of the immune system. The drug sodium chromalin used to prevent asthma attacks is a good example of how nutrients apply to medicine. The antiasthma drug was synthetically produced after research found that a plant flavonoid, khellin, prevents lung spasms.

Since many foodstuffs cause these allergies, hypoallergenic vitamins must be made synthetically, so as not contain any common allergens, such as soya, corn, wheat, milk, or eggs.

How Vitamins Can Protect Us against Pollution

In today's polluted world, vitamins can defend the system against toxic chemicals that insidiously find their way into our bodies from the air we breathe, the foods doused with acid rain and grown in pesticide-laden soils, and even the water we drink, which is laced with pollutants and toxic chemicals from industrial wastes.

Toxic chemicals have infiltrated every part of our lives. Apart from contamination with thousands of toxic chemicals, such as polychlorinated biphenyls (PCBS), oxides of nitrogen and sulfur, and acid-rain precipitates in the air, food additives and chemicals are found in everyday products. The FDA lists over 10,000 food additives. These are dyes in prepared foods, cosmetics, and drugs, as well as radioactive elements, such as radium, that silently attack our organs. Toxic gases leach from construction material, such as the formaldehyde gas used in insulation. All of these substances are known causes of diseases, cancer among them.

Estimates indicate that 90 percent of all human cancers can be attributed to environmental factors. Considering diseases such as cancer, which develop over a long period of time (from 1 to 20 years after exposure, or from persistent exposure), the use of vitamins as protection is an obvious answer, especially since the vitamins themselves act in a slow, continuous fashion.

Vitamins that specifically protect against damage from pollutants are called antioxidants, so named because they prevent oxidative processes. Scientific studies in the last decade have revealed that oxidative processes are involved in the formation of carcinomas. Many cancer-causing substances stimulate the production of free radicals (see chapter 13). Oxidant damage is also related to emphysema, atherosclerosis, ischemia, rheumatoid arthritis, cataracts, radiation injury, alcohol toxicity, and kidney damage from heavy metals.

The best-documented antioxidants against environmental pollutants are vitamins A, E, and C, and the minerals zinc and selenium. Scientific reports reveal that without a doubt vitamin E provides protection against damage to lungs caused by oxidants, specifically ozone and nitrogen dioxide in the atmosphere. Furthermore, vitamin E therapy has been found to give satisfactory results against respiratory distress (such as difficult breathing or wheezing, which is often associated with asthma).

Numerous tests have demonstrated that vitamin C is effective in protecting against liver damage caused by many environmental pollutants, as well as by alcohol and drugs such as acetaminophen, cocaine, and nicotine. Furthermore, vitamin C can reconvert oxidized vitamin E, thereby contributing a synergy that enhances the actions of vitamins and prolongs their lives within the body

Antioxidant vitamins and minerals are modern shields against the ravages of pollution. But be aware that in these tests, they were administered in megadoses or at levels exceeding the RDAS listed for each substance, indicating that their efficacy as pollution fighters depends on their concentration in the body. This scientific evidence has led the nutrition industry to develop combinations of antioxidants and high-dose vitamins for the seriously health-minded individual.

AMINO ACIDS

Amino acids are the building blocks of our cells. The proteins we eat break down to amino acids. Amino acids are essential to the proper function of all biosystems in our bodies. There are 22 amino acids, 14 that the human body can manufacture from the foods we eat and 8 that cannot be manufactured and must be provided in the diet, either from foods or from supplements. The 8 amino acids that the body cannot synthesize are frequently called essential amino acids, a rather misleading term, since all amino acids are essential to the generation and proper functioning of cells.

If the quantities of each amino acid, and their combinations, are incorrect, the new proteins, to be used for cellular reconstruction, will not be manufactured. If one amino acid in a specific chain is missing, protein synthesis may not occur at all, or it may occur only in proportion to the insufficiency. This can lead to infections, food and substance addiction, suppression of the immune system, allergies, stress, and symptoms of aging. Clearly, our everyday lives can be affected by amino acid deficiencies in many ways.

Amino acid deficiencies can also be caused by poor digestion of amino acids. The pancreas is the organ involved in breaking down proteins. The pancreatic enzyme that breaks down protein needs an alkaline medium to function. To establish this alkaline medium, the pancreas secretes bicarbonate. This allows the healthy production of the enzymes that break down protein. If there is not enough bicarbonate, these enzymes will be destroyed, resulting in lack of digestion of proteins and consequent multiple amino acid deficiencies. *Recent scientific research has found that amino acid deficiency is a major factor in such conditions as allergies, infections, and atherosclerosis, as well as in aging.*

How well amino acids metabolize will depend on the quality of the protein used to manufacture them. This is often determined by measuring the weight gain of an animal given a particular protein and is called the PER (Protein Efficiency Ratio). Many manufacturers of amino acids include the PER on the label.

Nitrogen balance is another way of determining protein quality. The United States Pharmacopeia has established a standard to measure the nitrogen balance for amino acid hydrolysates. The degree of breakdown (hydrolysis) is measured by the ratio between nitrogen from one amino acid (AN) to the nitrogen from the amino acid complex (TN). A value between 9 and 30 indicates a superior product. A value under 9 indicates that the protein has not been properly broken down. A value over 30 indicates that a high level of free amino acids is present. Reputable manufacturers include the AN/TN value on the label.

Product labels also describe amino acids as being either pure crystalline free-form amino acids (amino acids not connected in protein chains) or peptide-bonded amino acids (derived from foods or from the pancreatic digests of protein).

Absorption of amino acids occurs in the intestine and requires that peptides be present. Peptides are chains of amino acids rather than individual amino acids. They provide you with the optimum environment for total conversion of amino acids. In this form, the amino acids are balanced and ready to be absorbed by the bloodstream, and thus amino acid deficiencies are avoided. Peptide-bonded amino acids do not compete with each other for absorption, whereas pure crystalline free-form amino acids do, increasing the probability of deficiencies.

Research has shown free-form amino acids to cause diarrhea and anemia, as well as other major health problems. Hospital studies have indicated that peptide-bonded amino acids are more effective and better utilized by the body. Moreover, *pancreatic digests of protein have been used in nonallergenic infant formulae, as well as in speciality diets, for over 40 years.* And the medical profession prescribes pancreatic digests of protein to patients that have undergone bowel surgery.

Branched-Chain Amino Acids

You may see the letters BCAA on an amino acid product, most likely on a fuel pack for athletes. These letters stand for branched-chain amino acids. These are naturally occurring amino acids that provide a readily available source of fuel for the muscles as they are converted to blood sugar by the liver. This blood sugar (glucose) is used as fuel by muscles during workout. In general, such a product will be used to increase endurance and consequently performance. Branched-chain amino acids are used most by athletes. They are considered to be safe and without side effects by the health industry, but as with all amino acids, a nutrition expert should always be consulted before you use them.

Choosing Amino Acids

The important factors to consider in choosing amino acids are their methods of production, often indicated on the label, and the degree of hydrolysis. There are many methods of producing predigested proteins. The most common methods are:

−Using natural enzymes from plant or animal sources, which digest the proteins right in the living biosystem. These predigested proteins are then extracted.

−Using an acid to break down the protein.

−Using a base to break down the protein.

The best method is the natural-enzyme method, since it contributes compatible energy patterns from natural substances. Breaking down proteins with an acid or a base yields a high salt content and the production of toxic by-products, especially with the base.

The best amino acids are:

−Peptide-bonded and supplied by pancreatic digests of protein, rather than free-form amino acids. If labels claim that the amino acids are pharmaceutical-grade pancreatic digests, then they will be of top quality—providing the protein quality is optimal.

—From a good source and quality of protein, indicated by the PER or the AN/TN ratio on labels of reputable manufacturers.

Like many other health products, the best amino acid product is not necessarily the most expensive. In general, peptide-bonded amino acids from pancreatic digests of protein are less expensive than the less desirable pure crystalline free-form amino acids.

WHICH VITAMINS AND MINERALS ARE BEST FOR US?

The form of a vitamin, mineral, or amino acid also plays a role in the way the product will be assimilated by the body. Such effects begin as soon as the product is ingested. Capsules are much easier to swallow, and dissolve more quickly, than tablets, but because supplements are biochemically complex, the form in which they are taken affects how readily they are assimilated.

Dry Vitamins: Powder or Pure Crystalline

Dry vitamins are powdered, whereas pure crystalline vitamins appear as well-defined crystals under the electron microscope. The pure crystalline form is a synthetic, pharmaceutical product and is considered the purest form. When a pure crystalline powder is used for a vitamin, it is generally contained in a capsule, and no preservatives or other additives are included.

Vitamins are either fat soluble or water soluble. *Water-soluble vitamins are very easily absorbed and in fact pass almost directly into the bloodstream after they have been ingested.* Water-soluble vitamins are most often found in dry form, either as a powder or a pure crystalline form contained within a capsule or compressed into a tablet. The differences between the assimilation of tablets and capsules discussed in chapter 3 applies here. The less easily absorbed fat-soluble vitamins are usually in the form of gelules—soft gelatin capsules. Fat-soluble vitamins are oily, and the substance within the gelule is an oil. Fat-soluble vitamins can be broken up in water, usually resulting in an emulsion. Digestion, however, remains the same, and the fat-soluble vitamins must still bind with lipid molecules of bile salts in our bodies. Dry fat-soluble vitamins are less difficult to digest, because some of the excess oil is removed, and because they are broken up in water, so they can pass through the stomach and liver more easily. Dry fat-soluble vitamins are sold in powder form, usually in a hard gelatin capsule.

Vitamins in Liquid Form

There is a process that turns fat-soluble vitamins into water-soluble vitamins. The resulting vitamins are called micellized vitamins. Generally, micellized vitamins are so well assimilated by our bodies that their absorbency is magnified three- to four-fold. For example, a teaspoon containing about 400 ɪu or micellized vitamin E might act on the body as if 1600 ɪu of vitamin E were consumed. *Micellization is a recently developed process that gives us precious fat-soluble vitamins in liquid form that is very digestible and is excellent for older people with diminished digestive capacity or for young children and infants.*

Flavored Powders for Liquid Meal Replacements

Athletic supplements are aimed at body builders and serious athletes. Essentially, these products are amino acids and multi-supplements that combine vitamins with minerals, and sometimes herbs. More often than not, these products are in the form of powders, to be mixed with liquids and used as meal replacements. Meal replacements for dieters are made up mostly of amino acids, mainly because the lower the intake of calories, the greater the requirement of protein. Since protein breaks down into amino acids, a diet plan that provides readily available amino acids will provide sustenance while preserving precious energy. If amino acids are not supplied in a calorie-reduced diet, reserves of amino acids are used from body cells and tissues, causing wasting away—a very unhealthy way of losing weight!

Powders are more efficient than tablets or capsules because they are concentrates, which when reconstituted with beverages are then easily digested. Tablets and capsules, through, must first be broken down by digestion to release their active ingredients.

The table at the end of the chapter provides a quick reference of what to look for in each type of supplement.

Chelated Minerals

Chelation is a process that binds metals to amino acids. It is a complex chemical procedure that involves the forming of bonds, particularly covalent bonds and ionic bonds. These bonds are formed with the interaction between electrons and adjacent atoms. A covalent bond is very stable and requires a high temperature to be disrupted. Such a bond will prevent a mineral from being released too soon, when it would not be assimilated by the body. The electrons are also shared in ionic bonds, but the elements linked are electrolytes—conductors of electric currents. Many minerals are electrolytes, in particular, potassium, magnesium, and calcium. When dissolved in water, ionic bonds break down, releasing electrolytes. With supplements, the result is a mineral that will be easily broken down in the body and assimilated. Ionic and covalent bonds are what characterize a high-quality chelate. Unfortunately, whether chelates are covalent or ionic is rarely revealed on the labels of chelated minerals, but this information is beginning to appear in the manufacturers' product description and in some specialty magazines.

When an unchelated mineral enters the body, it must link up with an appropriate amino acid in order to be useful to cells.

Furthermore, if the amino acid required is deficient, cellular or tissue supplies will be used for chelation. *By taking an already chelated mineral, you are saving your body the energy it would require to bond that mineral with an amino acid, and preventing a potential amino acid deficiency.*

Mineral Complexes

Mineral complexes are minerals that are combined with acids from the Krebs cycle—a series of biochemical reactions that release energy for the cell to carry on its work. These minerals are usually recognized by a two-word complex, ending in "ate," such as calcium carbonate. There is scientific evidence that mineral complexes aid in the conversion of fat, carbohydrate, and protein into energy by carrying the mineral—which is necessary for so many enzyme reactions—right into the biochemical reaction. The Krebs cycle acid then acts as a kind of vehicle that swiftly ferries the mineral about. The mineral bound to a Krebs cycle acid can be thought of as wearing a pass in a restricted area, allowing it to enter freely. Scientific studies with athletes also show that mineral complexes reduce lactic acid buildup during performances. Lactic acid causes muscle spasms, excessive sweating, pain, and decreased endurance.

Biologically Formed Minerals

Biologically formed minerals are minerals that have been fed to brewer's yeast, whose cells incorporate the minerals in the same way as the cells in our bodies. These minerals are then extracted from the yeast and made into a supplement, usually in the form of a capsule or a tablet. The body readily assimilates these minerals because they are already in a form that can enter cells. Moreover, the minerals contribute the energy pattern acquired from being in the living biosystem of the yeast cells.

HOW VITAMINS WORK BEST

Vitamin	Most Effective When Taken With:	Antagonistic Substances	Causes of Deficiency
A	B-complex, C, E, D, calcium, phosphorus, zinc, some poly-unsaturated fatty acids (PUFA)	air pollution, alcohol, arsenicals (arsenic pollution), aspirin, corticosteroids, dicumarol, mineral oil, nitrates, phenobarbital, thyroid medicine	pollution, alcohol, certain diets
beta carotene	B-complex, C, D, calcium, zinc	same as for vitamin A	same as for vitamin A
B₁ (thiamine)	B-complex, B₂ (riboflavin), B₃ (niacin), folic acid, C, E, manganese, sulfur	alcohol, antibiotics, sugar dieting, nursing, preservatives, food processing	Caffeine, exercise, alcohol, pregnancy,
B₂ (riboflavin)	B-complex, B₃ (niacin), B₆, C	alcohol, antibiotics, oral contraceptives	alcohol, caffeine, physical activities, pregnancy, nursing, reducing diets
B₃ (niacin)	B-complex, B₁, B₂, C	alcohol, antibiotics, excess sugar	alcohol, caffeine, exercise, pregnancy, nursing, food processing, preservatives, heat

B$_5$ (pantothenic acid)	B-complex, B$_6$, B$_{12}$, C, biotin, folic acid, calcium, sulfur	aspirin, methylbromide (agricultural insecticide, residues on some foods)	alcohol, caffeine, exercise, pregnancy, nursing, reducing diets, food processing, heat
B$_6$ (pyridoxine)	B-complex, B$_1$, B$_2$, B$_5$, calcium, C, magnesium, potassium, linoleic acid, sodium	cortisone, estrogen, oral contraceptives	alcohol, caffeine, exercise, pregnancy, nursing, oral contraceptives, cooking of meat, reducing diets
B$_{12}$	B-complex, B$_6$, choline, inositol, folic acid, C, potassium, iron, sodium	dilantin, oral contraceptives nursing, vegetarian diet,	alcohol, caffeine, exercise, pregnancy,
biotin	B-complex, B$_2$, B$_5$, B$_6$, B$_{12}$, folic acid, niacin, C, sulfur	antibiotics, raw egg whites (avidin), sulfa drugs	sunlight, sleeping pills, reducing diets
C (ascorbic acid)	bioflavonoids, all vitamins and minerals	alcohol, antibiotics, antihistamines, aspirin, baking soda, barbituates, cortisone, DDT, estrogen, oral contraceptives, petroleum, sulfonamides, smoking	stress, pollution, oral contraceptives, water, cooking at high temperatures, light, smoking

Vitamin	Most Effective When Taken With:	Antagonistic Substances	Causes of Deficiency
choline	A, B-complex, B₁₂, folic acid, inositol, linoleic acid	alcohol, excess sugar	alcohol, food processing, pollution
D	A, C, choline, unsaturated fatty acids (UFA), calcium, phosphorus	alcohol, corticosteroid drugs, oral contraceptives, dilantin	mineral oil, alcohol, reducing diets
E	A, C, B-complex, inositol, B₁, unsaturated fatty acids, magesium, selenium	chlorine, inorganic iron, mineral oil, oral contraceptives, rancid fats and oils, antibiotics, air pollution	alcohol, caffeine, exercise, pregnancy, nursing heat, food processing, inorganic iron, chlorine, pollution
folic acid	B-complex, B₅, B₁₂, biotin, C	oral contraceptives, anticonvulsants, alcohol, phenobarbital	caffeine, alcohol, exercise, pregnancy nursing oral contraceptives, food processing, reducing diets
inositol	B-complex, B₁₂, choline, C, E, linoleic acid	antibiotics	pollution, preservatives, antibiotics, exercise
para-aminobenzoic acid (PABA)	B-complex, folic acid, C	sulfa drugs	smoking, pollution, sulfa drugs

	Most Effective When Taken With:	Antagonistic Substances	Causes of Deficiency
K	inconclusive information to date	air pollution, mineral oil, radiation, rancid oils and fats, anticoagulants	frozen foods, aspirin, air pollution, mineral oil, X rays
bioflavonoids (vitamin P)	C	alcohol, cortisone, insecticides	pollution, stress, antihistamines, smoking

HOW MINERALS WORK BEST

Minerals	*Most Effective When Taken With:*	*Antagonistic Substances*	*Causes of Deficiency*
calcium	A, C, D, iron (preferably time-released), unsaturated fatty acids, iron, magnesium, manganese, phosphorus, hydrochloric acid	aspirin, corticosteroid drugs, thyroid medicine	large quantities of fat, reducing diets
chromium	no conclusive information at this time	diet	reducing diets
cobalt	copper, iron, zinc	diet	pollution, smoking
copper	cobalt, iron, zinc	diet	menstruation, pregnancy, reducing diets

Minerals	Most Effective When Taken With:	Antagonistic Substances	Causes of Deficiency
iron	B_{12}, folic acid, C, calcium, cobalt, copper, phosphorus, hydrochloric acid	antacids, aspirin, EDTA (food preservative), E	alcohol, diuretics, reducing diets
magnesium	B_6, C, D, calcium, phosphorus, protein	alcohol, corticosteroid drugs, diuretics	reducing diets
manganese	B_1, E, calcium, phosphorus	antibiotics	caffeine, sugar, alcohol, reducing diets
phosphorus	A, D, unsaturated fatty acids, calcium, iron, manganese, protein	antacids, aspirin, corticosteroid drugs, diuretics, thyroid medicine	alcohol, smoking
potassium	B_6, sodium	aspirin, corticosteroid drugs, diuretics, sodium	food processing, large amounts of fat
selenium	E		pollution, smoking
zinc	A, B_6, E, calcium, copper, phosphorus	alcohol, corticosteroid drugs, diuretics, oral contraceptives	vegetarian diet, reducing diets

* The above represent only the more common vitamins and minerals. Some of the information in this table was taken from the second edition of the *Nutrition Almanac.*

FOR FURTHER READING

Chatham, M.; Eppler, J.; Sauder, L.; Green, D.; and Kulle, T. "Evaluation of the Effects of Vitamin C on Ozone-induced Bronchoconstriction in Normal Subjects." *Annals of the New York Academy of Sciences* 498 (1987).

Fletcher, B., and Tappel, A. "Protective Effects of Dietary Alphatocopherol in Rats Exposed to Toxic Levels of Ozone and Nitrogen Dioxide." *Environmental Research* 6 (1973).

Jensen, Bernard. "Chlorella: The Jewel of the East." *The Vitamin Supplement* (May 1988).

McGilvery, R. W. *Biochemistry: A Functional Approach.* Philadelphia, London, Toronto: W. B. Saunders Company, 1970.

Morrison, R. T., and Boyd, R. N. *Organic Chemistry.* Boston: Allyn and Bacon, 1973.

Philpott, W. H., and Kalita, D. K. *Brain Allergies: The Psycho-nutrient Connection.* New Canaan, Conn: Keats Publishing, 1980.

Pryor, W. A., ed. *Free Radicals in Biology.* New York: Academic Press, 1976.

Schoenkerman, B., and Justice, R. "Treatment of Allergic Diseases with a Combination of Antihistamine and Flavonoid." *Annals of Allergy* 10 (1952).

Silk, D. B. A., et al. "Comparison of Oral Feeding of Peptide and Amino Acid Mixtures to Normal Human Subjects." *Gut* 20 (1979).

Williams, Roger. *A Physician's Handbook on Orthomolecular Medicine.* New Canaan, Conn.: Keats Publishing, 1974.

TEN

Antistress Health Products

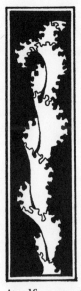

S tress is an insidious, intangible condition that causes very real physical ailments. Stress itself cannot inflict direct harm on the body or mind, but it can cause us to respond in ways that are deleterious to the nervous system, the emotions, and eventually to physiological processes. Given time, stress can ravage the body. *In fact, it has been clearly established that stress can provoke physical conditions that often lead to serious illness.* Most people recognize ulcers, migraines, and high blood pressure as stress induced, but such nagging minor ailments as muscle aches, constipation, and dermatitis can also signal the encroachment of stress.

Much of the power of stress lies in genetics, for genes contribute to the body's reaction to exterior forces. Stress attacks weak body areas first. If heart disease runs in your family, then you are predisposed to stress-induced heart conditions. If you sustained an injury as a child that weakened part of your musculoskeletal system, then stress may provoke rheumatism or arthritis, or simple muscular aches in that region of your body.

Stress works psychologically, irritating the emotions and implanting a feeling of helplessness. Scientists have studied this aspect of stress conclusively. This element of helplessness can be understood to relate to the natural healing principle that the physiological health of a biosystem depends on what surrounds its cells. When people feel they cannot control their lives, this feeling may lead to panic or despair. In time, this response will affect their bodies, and create negative changes in the cells' environment. Thus the physical effects of disease begin both at the energy level and at the cellular level.

STRESS IN PRIMITIVE AND MODERN TIMES

Understanding the genetic component of how we deal with stress leads us back to our primitive ancestors. The biology of the human metabolism during stress has not evolved. *Technology has changed our environment and our lives, but our metabolism has not adapted.* When primitive humans were faced with danger, as they were at almost every moment of their lives, physiological processes were mobilized, engaging the endocrine system to produce reactions that gave our primitive ancestors energy for a fighting chance against the forces of nature. When faced with danger, the body responds physiologically with a rise in blood pressure and the mobilization of endocrine and other autonomic processes that provide the "fight or flight" response necessary to deal with the danger.

In our modern society, the physiological processes mobilized by a strong emotional stimulus are usually not followed by action, but the endocrine and autonomic processes are still activated during stressful situations. The adrenal hormones make more sugar and fat available, and this surplus enabled our ancestors to respond with great physical effort. In modern life, the same metabolic changes occur in response to stress, but the sugar and fat mobilized is rarely used in physical effort. Instead the fat will be deposited in the lining of the arteries, predisposing us, and especially those that are genetically inclined, to heart conditions and other pathological conditions.

The interactions of our metabolic, psychological, and emotional states during stressful situations are so intimately connected that metabolic disturbances and disease can result from purely psychological stresses or psychosocial threats. For example, the blood levels obtained from oarsmen and their coach before and after a competitive race revealed that the same biochemical patterns occurred with psychosocial pressure, in the coach, as with physical pressure, in the oarsmen. After the race, the oarsmen showed a sharp decrease of white blood cells—a sign of physical stress. The white blood cell count of the coach, who sat in anxiety on the sidelines, was even lower than that of his oarsmen. This shows how *emotional stress can lead to the same metabolic effects as organic or physical stress.*

These observations can also be applied to laboratory animals, who are under a great deal of stress. And since science recognizes the harmful effects of stress, it should also be recognized that many tests involving laboratory animals cannot be conclusive, because all the subjects are under severe stress.

STAGES OF STRESS

According to famed stress expert Hans Selye, we adapt to stress in three stages: with an alarm reaction, a stage of resistance, and a stage of exhaustion.

During the alarm reaction of stress, the body produces corticoids, commonly called stress hormones. Experiments show that these hormones suppress our immune system.

During resistance, the body retaliates against the stress-induced reactions in the same way as it would against a drug in the biphasic reactions. According to stress researchers, the body uses any method to deal with the overload of hormones and their effects on the immune system. The results clearly show a chaotic situation in the body that can lead to diseases such as cancer.

During the exhaustion stage, our feeling of helplessness is

translated from the mental and emotional part of the biosystem to the physical part. The metabolic upheaval created in the biosystem causes exhaustion or metabolic breakdown, which occurs because the systems are in such disorder that they are unable to adapt. The results are physical ailments such as infections, viruses, flu, and so on.

The immune system seems to be the main link between stress and disease; probably because of the production of corticoids, which suppress the immune system at the onslaught of stress. Several scientific tests have revealed the disturbance of many body chemicals under stressful situations. One study of students' physical reactions to taking academic tests showed significant weakening of the immune system, as well as changes in protein, carbohydrate, and vitamin metabolism.

ANTISTRESS PRODUCTS

Today many products exist that claim to be stress fighters. Do they really suppress stress? And if they do, how do they work? Although there are many products that can alleviate symptoms or conditions triggered by stress, there is no product that can actually get rid of the source of the stress.

Researchers tell us that we can best manage stress by recognizing its symptoms and determining whether our physical or mental condition is caused by emotional stress or by such physiological problems as hormone imbalance or diet. This can be done with a medical examination and the use of such orthodox tests as blood tests, where necessary. If our symptoms are not the result of a physical condition, the identification of other stress factors can begin. Their management may include changing lifestyle and diet and practicing relaxation exercises. Experts in stress management warn you to incorporate these techniques gradually into your life, and that persistence is the key to success.

Health products advertised as "stress-busters" do have merit when they can alter the effects of stress by making the body more resistant. Most vitamins and nutrients can be thought of as stress fighters because they are involved in essential biochemical reactions, and are co-enzyme factors. Among other health products advertised as stress fighters are yeast-based tonics, amino acids, antianxiety nutrients, such as gamma amino butyric acid (GABA), and other nutrients, like inositol.

Liquid Yeast-Base Tonics

Yeast contains many nutrients and is particularly high in B vitamins and amino acids. The B vitamins build the blood and help make us more resistant to such ailments as anemia. For stress, yeast products could help someone predisposed to blood conditions but could negatively affect someone predisposed to yeast infections. Yeast also contains many amino acids, which are the basic building blocks of cells, but too many can bring the entire metabolism out of equilibrium, especially if the nutrients are not supplied in proper proportion.

Plasmolyzed yeast in contrast to plain yeast (see chapter 3) products, provide nutrients in well-balanced proportions, and with natural energy patterns. Research with plasmolyzed yeast products has revealed the positive influence such products have on the immune system. And if the immune system is able to resist stress, it will not so readily release harmful corticoids.

Amino Acids

Amino acid therapy is complex, and its discussion is beyond the scope of this book. However, many amino acid deficiencies have been linked to specific diseases. *Scientists are now finding that certain amino acids play an important role in stress management.* For example, tyrosine is a precursor norepinephrine, a chemical in the brain responsible for controlled behavior. Providing more tyrosine in the diet will yield more norepinephrine, and under stressful conditions, an abundance of norepinephrine will en-sure controlled behavior or response during high-stress mo-ments. When this hypothesis was tested on rats, researchers found that animals fed tyrosine-enriched diets were unaffected by stress, whereas rats on regular diets behaved abnormally.

Amino acid supplementation is an important new therapy, but stress management using only one amino acid to suppress a symptom does not treat the disease or the entire biosystem. Therapy with a number of amino acids, however, proportioned according to the person's metabolism, can become a useful con-tribution to a stress-fighting therapy.

Nutrients

GABA

Gamma amino butyric acid (GABA) is an amino acid derivative involved in complex reactions within the central nervous sys-tem. Within nutrition circles, GABA has been called an antiaging nutrient. In fact, GABA is an antianxiety nutrient. Studies have revealed that it has a calming effect, relieving anxiety and en-couraging sleep, making it a natural tranquilizer. There is evi-dence that this nutrient may also lower blood pressure. Like most nutrients, GABA works best synergistically with other nu-trients and vitamins, namely niacinamide and inositol.

DMAE

Dimethylaminoethanol (DMAE) is a natural amino alcohol, which is active in the brain. *DMAE is found naturally in sardines, herring, and anchovies.* Biochemically, DMAE is more of an antiaging nutrient, but the thin line that exists between the cel-lular reactions involved in stress mechanisms and the aging pro-cess makes this remarkable substance worth discussing. Dr. Hochschild, a researcher at the University of California, defines the leakage of enzymes from lysosomes (digestive structures found in cells that contain tissue-dissolving enzymes) as an aging process. He suggests that lysosomes are damaged by sex hormones, certain bacteria, free radicals and subsequent reactions, and radiation. If lysosomes are damaged, their lysosomal enzymes may leak into cells and surrounding connective tissue, resulting in damage to cell structures and in tissue breakdown. In biological terms, these are considered aging processes; however, they involve principles associated with stress. The influences of stress at the physiological level of the biosystem begin at the cellular level, causing biological stress. In this sense, DMAE is an antistress substance.

DMAE also breaks down nutrients from foods into more elemental products that the body can use and breaks down wastes into elemental components so that they are more easily excreted. It is important to note that this product requires specific preparation. Straight dimethylaminoethanol is alkaline and will burn the mucous membranes of the mouth and stomach. In short, it is a dangerous substance. However, the salt and the esters of this substance are used to prepare DMAE products. The product to look for in health food stores is the PABA salt of DMAE. This substance is a concentrated liquid that contains benzoic acid and potassium metabisulfide, which should be listed on the label.

Manufacturers represent DMAE as a safe natural brain stimulant. In a 1973 article by Dr. Hochschild in the journal *Experimental Gerontology,* DMAE was said to improve memory and learning, increase intelligence, elevate mood, and extend lifespan. But as with all remedies, a nutrition expert or holistic practitioner should be consulted for dosage and therapeutic use, and to ensure compatible interaction with any other remedies you may be taking.

Inositol

Inositol is a nutrient found in unprocessed whole grains, brewer's yeast, blackstrap molasses, liver, and citrus fruits. It reduces stress at the physiological level by sending oxygen to the tissues, enhancing the oxygen-binding capacity of hemoglobin.

Inositol mobilizes fat. Fat deposits in organs cause physiological stress by blocking the digestive system and consequently other systems. Furthermore, fatty infiltration of the liver taxes this organ and results in physical and mental fatigue. By guarding against these occurrences, inositol is an antistress substance.

Vitamins

PABA

Para-aminobenzoic acid (PABA) is a B vitamin. PABA's main value within the body is as a membrane stabilizer. It is closely related to DMAE in that it strengthens cellular membranes, preventing them from bursting and releasing dangerous lysosomal enzymes that will destroy surrounding tissue. In particular, PABA helps protect red blood cells. PABA may prevent our bodies from transforming certain amines into hallucinogenic drugs. In this respect, PABA *has been under investigation for its potential use in the treatment of mental conditions, such as schizophrenia.*

PABA generally comes in capsules. It is recognized by the health industry as a safe supplement. However, as with all remedies, a nutrition expert or holistic practitioner should be consulted for dosage and therapeutic use, and to ensure compatible interaction with any other remedies you may be taking.

Vitamin B_{12}

Vitamin B_{12} is also known as cobalamine or cyanocobalamine. Our bodies cannot synthesize B_{12}. It works as a stress fighter by regenerating red blood cells and thereby maintaining a healthy circulatory system. Moreover, B_{12} is necessary for the health of the nervous system and it decreases irritability—a definite by-product of stress.

Vitamin B_3

Vitamin B_3 is also known as niacin or niacinamide, and under its chemical name of nicotinic acid. It is found in poultry, lean meats, fish, and peanuts, and has been referred to as an antistress remedy because it brings on relaxation. But vitamin B_3 does more than give you a relaxed outlook. It reduces stress on the body by lowering cholesterol levels. In particular, niacin lowers the "bad cholesterol" known as LDL (low-density lipoproteins) and increases the "good cholesterol" known as HDL (high-density lipoproteins). Niacin also reduces the level of triglycerides in the blood; they are involved in the synthesis of VLDL (very low density lipoproteins)—the precursors to LDL. By removing and preventing the synthesis of these fat-containing bodies, niacin relieves the circulatory system of congestion, which would eventually tax other body systems and organs. In this respect, niacin reduces metabolic and physical stress.

Although niacin and niacinamide are similar, only niacin has a beneficial effect on the body's cholesterol. Unfortunately, niacin also brings a hot tingling feeling to the surface of the skin.

Vitamin B_5 (Pantothenic Acid)

Vitamin B_5 is found in brewer's yeast, whole-grain cereals, egg yolks, and organ meats. It is commonly referred to as an antistress vitamin because it plays a big part in keeping the adrenal glands healthy. The adrenal glands regulate metabolic functions. They produce cortisone and other hormones that regulate metabolic processes and thus directly affect the body's adaptability and its ability to withstand stress.

Vitamin B_6 (Pyridoxine)

Meat and whole grains are sources of vitamin B_6. It has many functions, but in relation to stress its most important role is in amino acid metabolism, because it helps our bodies to use amino acids from proteins. By helping the body use amino acids, vitamin B_6 relieves metabolic pressure and may be said to be an antistress vitamin.

Vitamin C (Ascorbic Acid)

When the body is under stress, the vitamin C normally contained in our adrenal glands is used up more quickly, and supplementation with this vitamin affects the body's ability to with-stand stress. Dr. Carl Pfeiffer, physician and author of *Mental and Elemental Nutrients,* has used vitamin C in the treatment of schizophrenia and claims that it has an antianxiety effect on the nervous system.

What is more relevant to stress, however, is that vitamin C restricts the production of corticoid hormones, which are nor-mally released during stressful situations. Because vitamin C suppresses the release of these corticoid hormones, it assists in the proper functioning of the immune system. In this light, we can say that *vitamin C gives the body greater resistance to stress.*

Several scientific studies have shown that stressful situations negatively affect our metabolism. Alterations in protein, carbo-hydrate, and vitamin metabolism, as well as depressed adrenal function, occur in people subjected to such stresses as academic testing. In some cases, just anticipating stressful situations can cause heart palpitations and changes in adrenal function. Any vitamin or mineral can be said to have an antistress effect on the body because it acts directly on the metabolism. However, tak-ing too many of these nutrients may also tax the metabolism by imposing too many molecules on it, leading to too many reac-tions.

All the above substances have been investigated scientifi-cally, and they are now used in stress therapy. However, there is no one "miracle" stress fighter. Most substances that contribute resistance to stress only work together with other substances and with appropriate management techniques.

ALLOPATHIC AND NATURAL ANTISTRESS REMEDIES

Since stress is an intangible entity seen in emotional and psy-chological states, as well as in physical reactions, there is no one substance that can annihilate it. Even relaxation exercises and body/mind exercises geared to relieve stress will not remove the stress. Any so-called antistress remedy, whether it is allopathic or natural or an exercise, will only remedy the symptoms. The main difference between allopathic and natural substances lies in their immediate and long-term effects. Allopathic drugs aim to treat only specific symptoms of stress. If the symptoms are psychological, such as anxiety, a tranquilizing drug such as Valium, or the commonly used phenothiazine will be prescribed. These substances calm the individual by sedation. But the biphasic effect will cause the body to fight the drug, and there may be many serious side effects, such as memory loss, fatigue, confusion, depression, headaches, and liver troubles. There is also increased anxiety when the medication is stopped, thereby creating emotional dependence on the drug.

In contrast, *a natural antistress substance will relieve symptoms of stress without inducing dependency or long-term side effects.* More important, it strengthens the organism and builds its resistance to stress. The stronger the organism, the less likely it is to be attacked by either microbes or stress. Moreover, the holistic approach tends to be more specific. Stress affects each individual in a different way. The metabolism of allopathic drugs often results in physical and metabolic ailments. For example, conventional antiulcer drugs usually work by reducing the secretion of gastric acid and pepsin. Prolonged use may cause amino acid deficiencies because protein is not adequately broken down and digested. Furthermore, these drugs may mask the symptoms of stomach cancer, diminishing the chances for early detection. Although dependence is low, these drugs can cause such side effects as confusion and dizziness.

Holistic remedies can be tailored to the individual. For example, homeopathic substances may be used to affect the emotional and psychological state of the patient. Other natural remedies, such as tinctures and herbs, can relieve such symptoms as anxiety, by acting the metabolism and readjusting the body's energy patterns. Furthermore, these remedies can act safely on the symptom, providing a tranquilizing effect, for example. But because of the information carried from the remedy's original biosystem, the natural tranquilizer will contribute more than just a tranquilizing effect.

Valerian *(Valeriana officinalis)* is a good example of how a natural substance can relieve tension while it primes the metabolism. Valerian is a plant that has been used as a tranquilizing agent and mixed with remedies to improve sleep. In fact, valerian should be marked as a stabilizing agent rather than a sedative. Pharmacologically, although valerian does indeed have sedative effects, scientific studies have shown that the valepotriates (substances in the plant that contribute the sedative effect) enhance the body's coordination and actually metabolically prevent the metabolism from fighting against this sedative effect. In this sense, the valepotriates balance the metabolism. In addition, they increase the power of concentration. *The mere balancing of the metabolism creates a calming effect on the individual.* If concentration is increased, one can function at greater capacity without experiencing undue stress. Moreover, valerian contributes symptomatic relief of physical ailments associated with anxiety, such as digestive spasms. Valerian contains a spasmolytic ingredient and an essential oil that is spasmolytic. For this reason, it is recommended to relieve and treat physical exhaustion, insomnia, and mental fatigue—all symptoms that can be associated with stress.

Holistic remedies relieve the physical symptoms of stress while they re-educate the metabolism to bring the organism to a state of wellness, naturally fostering greater resistance to stress. Allopathic drugs relieve surface symptoms, imposing long-term effects that burden the organism with a chain reaction of negative metabolic processes and psychological reactions.

FOR FURTHER READING

Canadian Medical Association. *Guide to Prescription and Over-the-Counter Drugs.* Montreal: Reader's Digest Association Canada, 1990.

Dubos, René. *Man Adapting.* New Haven and London: Yale University Press, 1965.

Driezen, S. "Nutrition and the Immune Response: A Review." *International Journal of Vitamin and Nutrition Research* 49 (1979).

Foley, D. "Clean out your Cholesterol." *Prevention* (July 1985).

Fritz-Niggli, Michel and Hedi. "The Influence of the Administration of a Yeast Preparation on the Radiation Syndrome in White Mice." *Hippokrates* 20 (1972).

Glaser, R., et al. "Stress-related Impairements in Cellular Immunity." *Psychiatry Research* 16 (1985).

Laudenslager, M. L., et al. "Coping and Immunosuppression: Inescapable But Not Escapable Shock Suppresses Lymphocyte Proliferation." *Science* (August 5, 1983).

Leibovitz, B. and Siegel, B. "Ascorbic Acid and the Immune Response." In *Diet and Resistance to Disease.* M. Phillips and A. Baetz eds. New York: Plenum Press, 1981.

Pearson, D. and Shaw, S. *Life Extensions.* New York: Warner Books, 1989.

Pfeiffer, Carl. *Mental and Elemental Nutrients: A Physician's Guide to Nutrition and Health Care.* New Canaan, Conn.: Keats Publishing, 1976.

Pharmaceutical profile and research literature from Vogel Laboratories, Switzerland, 1989.

Selye, H. *The Stress of Life.* New York: McGraw-Hill, 1976.

Shavit, Y. "Stress, Opioid Peptides, the Immune System, and Cancer." *Journal of Immunology* 135 (1985).

William, Roger. *Nutrition Against Disease.* New York: Pitman Publishing Co., 1971.

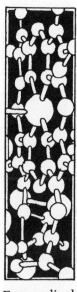

ELEVEN

Free Radicals

WHAT ARE FREE RADICALS?

Free radicals are atoms or molecules that contain an extra, unpaired electron, making them highly reactive and possibly damaging to cells in our bodies.

Free radicals are often the result of the oxidation or
peroxidation of polyunsaturated fatty acids. They are produced
in small amounts during normal metabolism, but they can also
arise from outside sources such as cigarette smoke, ozone, or insecticides, or as by-products during the metabolism of drugs,
pollutants, and such food additives as chemical dyes. They can
damage important molecules in our bodies, and they are implicated in the process of aging and a variety of diseases, such as
cancer, myocardial infarction, atherosclerosis, and rheumatoid
arthritis.

Free radical reactions are continuous; once they are produced, they create more free radical reactions, which continue
to generate free radicals. An example of the second law of entropy, free radicals are unruly and push the body into a state of
greater chaos.

WHERE ARE FREE RADICALS PRODUCED IN THE BODY?

Free radicals occur in the mitochondria, the lungs of the cell, where metabolized fuel is transformed into energy. They also occur in the endoplasmic reticulum, the membranes that metabolize foreign molecules, such as drugs.

Since free radicals are naturally produced in the body, they are sometimes useful. For instance, the immune system uses oxygen radicals to kill microbes. A study by Duwe, published in the *Journal of Immunology,* showed that natural killer cells, which are a class of white blood cell, use oxygen radicals to kill invaders. The study also revealed that the natural killer cells use this radical to destroy cancer cells. Unfortunately, the scavenging of free radicals does not end with invaders. These immune-generated radicals are very reactive and initiate another free radical reaction called lipid peroxidation. When this happens, DNA, proteins, and other molecules are damaged, leading to irreversible damage of tissues.

Free radicals are responsible for the painful inflammation of rheumatoid arthritis. They cause the breakdown of hyaluronic acid, the substance that protects joints from mechanical damage, acting like a glue to prevent the spread of viruses. This is how the vicious cycle continues. The free radicals are generated, then they go on to produce more free radical reactions, then some of the free radicals start breaking down healthy tissue to cause permanent damage.

In a study by Hewitt and colleagues, cellular examination revealed that inflamed arthritic tissue was characterized by fluorescence, which is associated with the pigment lipofuscin, generated as a result of free radical damage. The pigment lipofuscin is known as the "age pigment" and is commonly seen as brown spots that appear on the skin of aging individuals. It is used to determine a person's biological age—the extent of wear on the internal body.

Free radicals also attract other harmful substances that in turn cause entropy or direct damage to cells and irreversible damage to tissues. For example, the presence of free radicals sets the stage for cancer by decreasing immunity and by decreasing the fluidity of cell membranes, thus interfering with the passage of essential ions. The inevitable increase in free radicals moving through the body attracts harmful chemicals. Nitrites, for example, are transformed into their reactive or "proximate" state, as nitrosamines. Free radicals are directly involved in cancer, since they are linked to both the initiation phase of cancer, when cells are altered, and to the promoter stage of cancer, when damaged cells mutate and multiply and chemicals are transformed from their noncarcinogenic (harmless) state to their carcinogenic (cancer-causing) state.

QUENCHING FREE RADICALS

Free radicals can be neutralized naturally in the body by specific enzymes, or by antioxidants. In the body, there are four enzymes that essentially defuse free radicals: superoxide dismutase (SOD), glutathione peroxidase (GSH Px), S-tranferase, and catalase.

SOD is found naturally in all cells that use oxygen, and as such it detoxifies oxygen radicals known as superoxide radicals (SOR). *Superoxide dismutase has been marketed as a nutrient that defuses free radicals. In reality, SOD taken orally is broken down and rendered inactive by the gastrointestinal tract.* In clinical trials, SOD has been injected as a potential cure of certain diseases, but even in injectable form SOD is not very stable and survives only a short time in the bloodstream. However, the minerals zinc and copper and sometimes manganese are components of superoxide dismutase, so adding these minerals to the diet will increase the natural production of superoxide dismutase.

GSH Px defuses a number of free radical reactions. Because a major component of this enzyme is the trace mineral selenium, it is possible to increase GSH Px production within the body with selenium supplements. L-glutathione is also a component of GSH Px. L-glutathione is itself composed of cysteine, glutamic acid, and glycine, and activates another group of antioxidant enzymes called S-transferases. By taking the amino acids cysteine, glycine, and glutamic acid, or L-glutathione, you are providing your body with the ingredients necessary to naturally manufacture S-transferase.

S-transferase binds with foreign molecules, removing them from the system.

Catalase detoxifies certain free radicals but seems to be less important than superoxide dismutase and glutathione peroxidase.

ANTIOXIDANTS AGAINST FREE RADICALS

As already mentioned, some vitamins, such as A and E, are antioxidants. Any antioxidant vitamin or nutrient will scavenge or "quench" free radicals.

You may wonder about destroying free radicals, since some of them scavenge such unwanted foreign molecules as microbes in our bodies. The problem is that these initially good reactions produce more free radical reactions that in turn produce more free radicals. When this happens, there are too many free radicals floating around the body with nothing to attack. So instead, they damage healthy cells and tissues. Supplementation with antioxidant vitamins will scavenge those free-floating radicals, but not the initial microbe fighters.

If you live in a polluted area, or eat many fatty foods, you are likely to generate a higher ratio of free radicals than those who live in a relatively unpolluted area and are careful about what they put into their bodies. Where there is a good equilibrium, the body will maintain itself. But in this day and age, everyone should consume antioxidants, though some will require more than others, because of their lifestyle and diet. A health professional should always be consulted for specific therapy.

Certain nutrients provoke free radicals. For example, iron has been used in the laboratory to create free radical reactions. In a 1988 study reported in the *New England Journal of Medicine*, 14,000 adults were followed for a period of thirteen years. Men with high iron levels were five times more prone to develop cancer of the colon than men with low iron levels. An animal study has demonstrated that iron overload also promotes tumor growth in animals.

COMBINING ANTIOXIDANTS

To date, research offers much evidence that compared with the effects of single uses, combining antioxidants offers greater protection against free radical damage. There is evidence to suggest that antioxidants work together to protect cells and tissues and to protect each other from oxidation (transformation by oxygen). For example, vitamin E protects beta carotene and vitamin A (retinol) from oxidation. It also prevents oxidation of cell membranes, thus preventing them from rupturing and spilling enzymes that can destroy tissue. *Vitamin C reconverts oxidized vitamin E to its protective form, reduced tocopherol.* Beta carotene deactivates free radicals.

A 1987 study published in *Cancer Research* demonstrated that when vitamin E was given along with glutathione and selenium, it was 20 percent more effective at reducing tumor formation than when given alone. Other studies have shown that vitamins C and E and glutathione given in combinations were more effective at inhibiting a certain type of free radical reaction than when these nutrients were given alone. Evidence also suggests that coenzyme Q_{10}, a natural nutrient present in human heart muscle and available in such foods as corn and soybean oils, fish, chicken, nuts, and rice bran, combined with vitamin E is highly effective in fighting free radicals.

Thus, it is clear that antioxidant nutrients are best taken in combination. Copper, zinc, and manganese are needed to produce SOD within the body. Another important antioxidant enzyme requires selenium and the amino acid cysteine, which is found in wheat germ, poultry, and ham. It may also be taken as a supplement in capsule, tablet, or powdered form. For further protection, beta carotene, vitamin E, selenium, and vitamin C should also be taken.

FOR FURTHER READING

Armstrong, D.; Sohal, R. S.; Cutler, R.; and Slater, T., eds. *Free Radicals in Molecular Biology, Aging and Disease*. New York: Raven Press, 1984.

Bendich, A. et al. "Interaction of Dietary Vitamin C and Vitamin E in Guinea Pig Immune Responses to Mitogens." *Journal of Nutrition* 114 (1984).

Duwe, A. K. et al. "Natural Killer Cell-mediated Lysis Involves an Hydroxyl Radical-dependent Step." *Journal of Immunology* 134 (1985).

Hewitt, S.; Lunec, J.; Morris, C; and Blake, D. "Effect of Free Radical-altered IgG on Allergic Inflammation." *Annals of Rheumatic Disease* 46 (1987).

Horvath, P., and Ip, C. "Synergistic Effect of Vitamin E and Selenium in the Chemoprevention of Mammary Carcinogenesis in Rats." *Cancer Research* 43 (1983).

Leibovitz, B., and Siegel, B. V. "Aspects of Free Radical Reactions in Biological Systems Aging." *Journal of Gerontology* 35 (1980).

Leung, H., and Morrow, P. "Interaction of Glutathione and Ascorbic Acid in Guinea Pig Lungs Exposed to Nitrogen Dioxide." *Research Communications in Chemical Pathology and Pharmacology* 31 (1981).

Machlin, L. J., and Bendich, A. "Free Radical Tissue Damage: Protective Role of Antioxidant Nutrients." *Federation of American Societies for Experimental Biology Journal* 1 (1987).

Perchellet, J. P. et al. "Effects of Combined Treatments with Selenium, Glutathione, and Vitamin E on Glutathione Peroxidase Activity, Ornithine Decarboxylase Induction, and Complete and Multistage Carcinogenesis in Mouse Skin." *Cancer Research* 47 (1987).

Pryor, W., ed. *Free Radicals in Biology.* Vol. VI. Orlando, Fla.: Academic Press, 1984.

Stevens, R.; Jones, Y.; Micozzi, M.; and Taylor, P. "Body Iron Stores and the Risk of Cancer." *New England Journal of Medicine* 319 (1988).

Weinberg, E. "Iron in Neoplastic Disease." *Nutrition and Cancer* 4 (1983).

Zidenberg-Cherr, S.; Keen, C.; Lonnerdal, B.; and Hurley, L. "Dietary Superoxide Dismutase Does Not Affect Tissue Levels." *American Journal of Clinical Nutrition* 37 (1983).

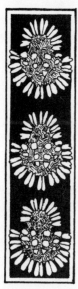

TWELVE

Natural Remedies
for Health Crises

Many natural substances and nutrients have been studied and are now used therapeutically for a variety of conditions by both allopathic and holistic medical practitioners. The following page describe a number of remedies for specific ailments and situations.

PREPARING FOR HOSPITAL

Before specific ailments are dealt with, it is interesting to note that more and more allopathic physicians are using nutrients to prepare their patients for surgery. Moreover, many other *physicians promote the use of herbal remedies and nutrients as postsurgical remedies to speed recovery.* For example, Dr. V. Hufnagel, author of *No More Hysterectomies,* puts her patients on amino acids before and after surgery. She works with biochemists and nutritionists to help find the proper combinations of nutrients to fuel recovery processes specific to various types of surgery.

It is important to supplement amino acids during illness, and before and after surgery. Several research physicians report grave amino acid deficiencies in their patients after hospitalization or surgery. When the body is under stress, whether physical or mental, amino acids are mobilized and used by the liver to make glucose. This biochemical reaction quickly results in amino acid deficiencies. Eventually, the immune system fails because amino acids are not available to form antibodies. When there is no amino acid supplementation, the amino acids used up by the body also cause severe weight loss.

Often hospital routines further exacerbate amino acid deficiency. According to one medical researcher, amino acid malnutrition is increased by the dextrose intravenous feeding commonly used with seriously ill patients. Moreover, hospital food is overcooked and depleted of natural vitamins and amino acids.

Another nutrient highly recommended by allopathic practitioners is vitamin C, mainly because it regulates stress reactions by suppressing immune hormones and increasing the activity of phagocytes—the cells that eat pathogens. In this way, vitamin C helps the body to recovery and to resist stress. Some physicians prescribe over 3 grams of vitamin C for pre- and post-surgical therapy.

More and more, allopathic doctors are joining the ranks of holistic doctors in prescribing antioxidants before and after surgery to diminish the harmful effects of anesthetic drugs. Specifically, beta carotene, vitamin E (usually in its easily digestible dry form), glutathione, N-acetyl cysteine, zinc, and synthetic selenium (selenate) are recommended. Vitamin C may also be used.

An article in the *American Journal of Clinical Nutrition* revealed that zinc is more available to the biosystem if it is bound to picolinic acid, forming zinc picolinate. The article suggests that zinc picolinate is more readily and efficiently absorbed than the more common zinc gluconate or zinc citrate. Moreover, another complex known as zinc histidine was found to be so well absorbed that only 15 milligrams of zinc histidine complex was needed to yield an equal level of zinc in the bloodstream as 45 milligrams of zinc sulfate. However, *any form of zinc will enhance the function of the immune system*. Specifically, zinc regulates the thymus gland, which "tells" T-cells what to do. When the thymus gland is under stress, such as during illness, the T-cell function will be diminished. Moreover, as we age, the thymus gland shrinks and T-cell activity diminishes. In fact, one study revealed that T-cell function was restored in deficient animals by zinc supplementation. In short, *as zinc is not readily available in the foods we eat, supplementing 10 to 15 milligrams a day is a good idea.*

OTHER HOLISTIC WAYS TO HELP REMOVE TOXINS

Herbal teas are an excellent way to flush your system of toxins after surgery. The specific herb can be chosen in accordance with the body part to be healed. For example, dandelion tea is used to detoxify the liver. Remember that the active principle contained in the tea is in too low a concentration to be fully therapeutic. However, drinking two to three cups a day disperses the active principles of the tea throughout the body, together with a good amount of water, which will help flush the system. Herbal tea is probably safer than taking diuretic herbal capsules after surgery, because your system is already under enough stress and you do not want to cause entropy. The digestive organs, particularly the liver and the kidneys, are under enormous stress after surgery. So take herbal remedies in liquid form to reinforce these organs or to help them rid your body of toxins. The active ingredients of a herbal liquid require little digestion before entering the bloodstream and thus will not stress the organs. Thus, for one to two weeks after surgery, take extracts, tinctures, teas, or essential oils rather than dried, or even lyophilized, capsules. Reserve the capsules for later—about 10 days after surgery.

Plasmolyzed yeast solutions are excellent tonics after surgery or during any type of convalescence. They provide the body not only with herbal principles but also with a balanced amount of amino acids. Plasmolyzed yeast solutions are made by feeding fresh organic herbs to yeast cells, which incorporate the plants' principles. The contents of the cells are then exploded (plasmolyzed), and their extraneous membranes are removed by straining. The resultant solution is essentially the contents of a "whole" biosystem. The yeast cell contains protein (amino acids), carbohydrates, fats, enzymes, vitamins, and minerals, and the herbs contain substances that have specific effects on the physical organs and on their function within the body. This "whole" substance therefore benefits the body in every respect. Experiments in England revealed that plasmolyzed yeast tonic increased the activity of the liver enzyme, thereby increasing the body's ability to break down foreign substances found in anesthetic drugs. A Swiss double-blind study found that *plasmolyzed yeast significantly enhanced the ability of the blood protein hemoglobin to carry oxygen to the tissues. It also enhanced appetite, body weight, and recovery rate, and protected patients against radiation toxicity.*

Similar results were found with chlorella extracts. Chlorella provides an alternative to plasmolyzed yeast for those who have yeast intolerance. Liquid chlorella is available, but it is quite expensive.

REMEDIES FOR SPECIFIC AILMENTS

The Common Cold or Flu

There is still no cure for the common cold. Allopathic medicine offers many remedies for cold or flu symptoms but nothing to reinforce the system and help it recover. Holistic medicine, in contrast, provides a variety of soothing natural remedies that boost the immune system and enhance physiological functions, as well as providing relief from symptoms. Moreover, there are homeopathic dilutions for the flu, but these must be prescribed by a homeopathic physician.

Herbal Remedies for Colds and Flu

Extract or tincture of goldenrod *(Solidago Virga auren)* relieves pain and eliminates toxins because of its diuretic effect. It is also an astringent for the intestine, which is helpful when diarrhea accompanies the flu.

A homeopathic dilution of bryonia *(Bryonia dioica)* relieves inflammation of the mucous membranes, which includes sore nasal passages due to sniffles and blowing your nose, as well as inflamed bronchial membranes in cases of bronchitis. Bryonia also helps thin and expectorate mucus.

A homeopathic dilution of aconite *(Aconitum napellus)* helps relieve fever, especially at its onset. It also helps calm palpitations of the heart, which are common to colds and flu when the body is under so much physical stress.

Extract or tincture of baptisia *(Baptisia leucantha)* is another herbal remedy that cuts fever. Traditionally, it is used in homeopathic dilutions. It is a general tonic for exhaustion and thus can provide adjuvant therapy for colds and flu. It also has anti-infection capacity.

Extract or tincture of oat *(Avena sativa)* provides a toniclike quality when you are sick with the cold or flu. Specifically, it contributes vitamins A, B, and D and bioflavonoids, and helps prevent dehydration. *Oat extract relaxes the body, allowing you to rest.*

Extract or tincture of purple cone flower *(Echinacea purpurea)* is a great immune booster. It stimulates the production of interferon, a natural antibiotic. Moreover, it contains the B factor, which inhibits hyaluronidase, an enzyme that thins the gluelike material between cells, and thus prevents the spread of microorganisms, viruses, and other toxins throughout the body. European studies have shown that purple cone flower increases the activity of white blood cells. *Purple cone flower is especially effective for infections of the respiratory system and also an indispensable immune booster during any illness.*

Garlic and onions have over 75 sulfur-containing sub-stances, some of which are natural antibiotics. Onions contain a high amount of a bioflavonoid, quercitin—a potent deconges-tant. Studies have shown that both garlic and onions have anti-bacterial properties. They are known to kill *Clostridium pseudo-monas* and *Salmonella* bacteria. Eating garlic and onions raw, or consuming the essential oil of garlic or onion, will contribute these properties. There are garlic and onion capsules that do not have any odor. The choice is yours.

Essential oil of clove is a potent virus fighter. You must exer-cise caution when using this essential oil, since it is a phenol and is potentially neurotoxic. It must not be given to pregnant women, as it will induce labour. Two or three drops in honey is all that is needed to help rid the system of the cold virus. When using essential oils, always consult a health professional.

Food for Your Cold

Many foods are recommended during illness. Although the ef-fectiveness of most of these is based on superstition, the effica-cious ones have chemicals that lend therapeutic properties. Chicken soup is a good example. Many swear by its "miracu-lous" curative powers, especially for colds or flu. Dr. Joseph Vitale of the Boston University School of Medicine believes that hot, steaming remedies like tea and chicken soup help because the steam loosens mucus, thereby decongesting and helping to expel infectious microorganisms. But *chicken soup also contains a great deal of ornithine—an amino acid implicated in the proper func-tioning of the immune system.* Researchers at Albert Einstein Col-lege of Medicine have shown that ornithine assists in post injury healing by repairing collagen and that it also stimulates the re-lease of Growth Hormone (GH), which is necessary for the proper functioning of the immune system. In addition, they found that arginine supplements (arginine is an amino acid that converts naturally to ornithine in our bodies) increase the activ-ity and size of the thymus gland, which regulates the activity of the T-cells, which destroy viruses, bacteria, and tumors. Other studies reveal that among other things, ornithine and arginine enhance the liver function, protecting against mental fatigue if the liver malfunctions. Homemade chicken soup is naturally abundant in ornithine and arginine, illustrating how foods can be good medicine.

Remedies to Help Thin Mucus and Help Relieve Stuffiness

Mexicans tell you how you can clear your sinuses with seasonings, such as cayenne, paprika, and horseradish. Many allopathic physicians recommend putting horseradish in honey to help relieve stuffy nose, throat, and lungs. In fact, there are many natural herbal remedies made with tincture of horseradish to relieve stuffiness.

Cough Remedies

To help thin the mucus and reduce the spasms of cough, essential oil of rosemary *(Rosmarinus officinalis)* is quite effective. Ipecac also has long been reputed to increase secretion and liquefication of mucus. Although ipecac is also an irritant used to induce vomiting in children, it is quite effective in the proper dilution in herbal cough mixtures. The extract of English Ivy *(Hedera helix)* leaves is also used as an expectorant and antispasmodic, especially for dry, spastic coughs.

You will often find pine juice in cough remedies. Pine juice made from the shoots contains essential oils, resins, sugars, and vitamin C. It has long been reputed as both a cough sedative and an expectorant. Generally, two dropperfuls of tincture are used per cup of honey. The specific proportions depend on the tincture or extract. For complete accuracy, consult a herbalist or natural pharmacist.

To make a cough syrup with any of these herbs, you simply add a tincture or an extract of the herb to unpasteurized honey. (But note that unpasteurized honey can be fatal to babies.)

Other Cold Decongestants

Vitamin C has been touted as a cold remedy that will stop your cold, but vitamin C will not destroy the cold virus. However, it is antihistaminic and will decongest your lungs, nose, and throat quite efficiently. Large doses of chewable vitamin C are preferable because chewable vitamin C usually contains calcium, which buffers the acid. In addition, the chewable form is partially digested by enzymes in the mouth and absorbed through the mucous membranes, fragmenting the dosage and allowing the vitamin's decongestant action to take immediate effect.

Zinc is another excellent remedy. It will prevent colds by fortifying the immune system, since it stimulates the activity of T-cells. Studies have shown that diets supplemented with zinc restore normal function of T-cells in deficient animals. Besides these immune system benefits, zinc will relieve many symptoms of a cold, such as sore throat, ringing in the ears, and a sore, runny nose.

A few drops of essential oil of lavender (**Lavandula vera**) *placed on a handkerchief will act as a decongestant inhaler.* Do not take this oil internally, however, as it is not effective in this form.

Extract of ephedra *(Ephedra sinica)*, a Chinese plant, is a potent decongestant, recommended for daytime relief of congestion, since it does not induce drowsiness.

Nerve Remedies

Many remedies and nutrients that benefit the nervous system are discussed throughout this book. When looking for a prepared remedy for the nerves, you are basically looking for something to help reduce or manage your stress level. Chapter 10 is devoted to natural remedies and stress.

Apart from this, a nerve remedy should be a nerve tonic. It should contain a substance to relax the biosystem, such as oat extract or niacin. Oat extract might be the better choice, because it contains vitamins A, B, and D and bioflavonoids that act as an adjuvant therapy on the biosystem.

Oat extract might also contain an amino acid or a combination that could restore proper balance to the biosystem. Such amino acids as glutamine act specifically on the mental-emotional level. This substance is one of the few substances that are able to pass the blood-brain barrier, a protective barrier of the brain that is very selective about the substances it allows to cross into the brain.

Insomnia Remedies

Insomnia may be a secondary reaction to stress. If so, stress management will be necessary to cure it. A good remedy against insomnia, however, contains a natural sedative, an antispasmodic, and a tranquilizing agent that works by increasing concentration and proper functioning of the brain and body. Valerian has this kind of equilibrating effect. Valerian contains valepotriates, and experiments with these substances reveal increased coordination of the body rather than a hypnotic effect. Added to extract of hops, containing lupulin, which is antispasmodic, antihistaminic, and mildly sedative, they make a good remedy for insomnia.

Let us not forget the most popular herbal "relaxing" remedy, passionflower *(Passiflora incarnata)* extract and melissa *(Melissa officinalis)*. Experiments have demonstrated the sedative and antispasmodic effects of passionflower. It is particularly useful in cases of nervous strain or stress, and works best as a daytime sedative. Melissa extract and essential oil of melissa are effective as antispasmodics.

Natural Remedies for Menstrual Difficulties

Menstrual difficulties can result from many problems. They can be caused by hormonal imbalance, injury, stress, and so on.

Specific diagnosis from a specialist should always precede any type of treatment.

If hormonal therapy is required, there may be some natural alternatives. Since the hypothalamus, pituitary, thyroid, and adrenal glands and the ovaries control hormone levels, herbals or nutrients that influence these glands are called for. Thus Dr. Hufnagel uses a combination of amino acids to regulate certain hormonally induced menstrual problems.

Glandular tissue extracts are also commercially available. These are homeopathic remedies made from biological tissue extracts and are used to stimulate the affected gland. Of course, they should not be experimented with and require prescription by a specialist who is also a homeopathic physician.

Nutrients like zinc and vitamin C help to keep the integrity of the reproductive system intact. Vitamin E is helpful for premenstrual syndrome but must be taken in large doses of 700 iu and up to be effective. B_6 has been used by European doctors for years to prevent morning sickness, and it has proved useful in controlling some of the symptoms associated with pms.

Sepia is a homeopathic remedy extracted from cuttlefish that has been used for decades by European homeopaths as a gynecological remedy. It is effective in treating exhaustion associated with menstrual difficulties. After the sepia is extracted from the cuttlefish, it is made into a homeopathic dilution. This dilution is recommended for regulating the menstrual cycle and for such associated symptoms as nervous exhaustion, irritability, cramps, insomnia, and pain in the lumbar area.

Prostate Remedies

A good prostate remedy should be decongestant, antispasmodic, and antiphlogistic, and many herbs fulfil these needs. Sabal *(Sabal serratata)* works as a decongestant to the edema caused in prostate conditions. Poplar *(Populus tremula)* is a potent antispasmodic and has been used by European doctors for the painful urination commonly associated with prostate problems.

The mineral zinc has long been recognized as the "male mineral" because of its usefulness in the treatment of prostate conditions. Allopathic doctors regularly recommend zinc for prostate conditions.

A Natural Laxative

An efficient laxative needs adjuvant therapy to cope with the other reactions due to constipation, such as liver congestion, toxicity, inflammation and irritation of the lining of the intestine, decreased appetite, and decreased movement of the intestine.

Most natural laxatives contain senna *(Cassia angustifolia)*. This herb is chosen because it contains a glycoside whose aglycone becomes active only when it reaches the intestine under the influence of the bacterial flora. The bacterial flora causes the glycoside to split, releasing anthraquinones (anthron or dianthron glycosides), which stimulate movement of the intestine. The result is agitation of the bacterial flora, which breaks down the contents of the intestine.

Many people complain that natural laxatives take a long time to work. This is because breakdown of the active principles occurs in the intestine. Moreover, *a laxative must act slowly so as not to shock the system.* With senna, the reaction leading to agitation of the bacterial flora occurs 8 to 10 hours after ingestion.

An adjuvant to such a good "agitator" as senna contains an agent to stimulate or decongest the liver, such as dandelion and chicory. Dandelion contains bitters that stimulate digestion. Chicory *(Taraxacum officinalis)* contains vitamin A, B, C, and K and bioflavonoids, making it useful in cases of vitamin deficiency. This often is a secondary reaction to constipation, because the system is upset, not eliminating and therefore not absorbing. *Fennel* **(Foeniculum vulgare)** *is a useful addition to a laxative remedy as it is an antispasmodic agent, especially in the stom-*

ach, but encourages movement in the intestine. Fennel is also antiflatulent and stimulates the liver.

Finally, some type of mucilaginous fiber would work to soften stool and facilitate elimination. Buckthorn *(Rhamnus cathartica)* is a good choice, since it also stimulates the gallbladder and as such acts as an adjuvant. Contrary to popular belief, fiber does not cause diarrhea and is not really a laxative. Fiber regulates elimination by regulating stool volume and transit time. Insoluble fiber such as cellulose may relieve constipation by causing bulking action.

Most natural laxatives contain a combination of these ingredients and may appear as tablets or liquids. Such natural laxatives are not habit forming and can be safely effective when necessary. But a sound diet with a high fiber content is always preferred to any type of remedy.

Remedies for Diarrhea

Medicinal clay, which can be white, gray, red, or green natural clay mud, is collected and placed in a pyramidlike container, where it is dried in the sun. This container is specially designed so that the clay can absorb energy from the sun. Medicinal clay is useful for different ailments, depending on its color. Gray clay coats and soothes irritated mucosa. Moreover, clay will capture toxins that may be causing diarrhea and carry them safely out of the body. Medicinal clay is available at health food stores and is a safe remedy for internal applications.

Extract of the root of the tormentil plant *(Potentilla tormentilla)* has commonly been used to treat diarrhea. It contains many tannins, which are natural astringents. These astringents will check inflammation of both the stomach and intestinal linings.

The use of loosestrife *(Lythrum salicaria)* date back to antiquity. Dioskurides recommended it for dysentery, and others as a cure for diarrhea. In pharmacy it is recognized as an astringent.

Knotweed *(Polygonum aviculare)* is another extract used by conventional medicine to treat diarrhea as well as the symptoms of dysentery. It contains about 4 percent tannin.

Most remedies for diarrhea contain a combination of the ingredients discussed or may contain only one strongly astringent plant extract like tormentil root extract or wild strawberry *(Fragaria vesca)* extract. Although these remedies are safe for simple cases of diarrhea, it is always important to consult a physician, as diarrhea is often associated with other, more serious illnesses.

Remedies for Cuts, Scrapes, and Burns

Juice or gel of aloe vera is recommended for cuts, scrapes, and burns. Aloe vera is anti-inflammatory, antibacterial, and antifungal, and promotes the regeneration of skin cells. But beware, because not all aloe products are created equal. To have medicinal properties, the aloe vera plant must be at least four years old. Some products contain additives that counteract the effects of aloe vera. For instance, potassium benzoate may irritate the skin. Look for aloe products that contain no additives or that contain natural ingredients such as vitamin C, which acts as a natural preservative as a result of its antioxidant properties. Many companies tout these "natural preservatives" on their labels.

A Remedy for the Liver

A feeling of nausea, difficult digestion, and constipation, combined with acne-type breakouts and tiredness, especially after meals, may indicate a sluggish liver. Most remedies for the liver aim to increase the secretion of bile. The best-known active substance, silymarin, is actually a flavonoside from the thistle *(Silybum marianum)* seed. Silymarin's action has been known for a long time, and Mayer and Menge in 1949 reported good clinical results in treating hepatitis with it. Other studies revealed that thistle protects the liver against the toxic molecules in pharmaceutical drugs. But it was only in 1968 that it was identified as acting to protect the liver.

Artichoke *(Cynara scolymus)* is another liver remedy that has been touted for years as a bile stimulant. Like thistle, artichoke extract can increase the flow of bile by 60 percent.

Tamarind is a spice that comes from the fruit of the tamarinacea *(Tamarindus indica)* tree. In Europe it has been used for centuries as a remedy to stimulate liver and gallbladder function.

Dandelion is a very efficacious bile stimulant. It relieves the sensation of bloating and nausea very quickly, and cleanses the liver.

Natural formulae to improve digestion by the liver usually contain a combination of extracts with high concentrations of bile stimulants like the ones discussed. Although natural remedies are deemed safe by the health industry, it is important to consult a physician for liver ailments, since these disturbances are often associated with more serious illnesses.

Remedies to Improve Digestion

Bitters are the most widely used natural substances to increase appetite and improve digestion. Most wild plants contain bitters. Peruvian bark *(Cinchona succirubra)* is commonly used as a strong bitter to stimulate gastric juices. The plant sweet flag *(Acorus calamus)* also contains bitters and useful and safe essential oils that help the appetite and digestion, and it also relieves cramps. The most popular natural remedy for indigestion is gentian yellow *(Gentiana lutea)*. Europeans make wine and other liqueurs with this medicinal plant. Gentian yellow is unique in containing bitters that remain potent even when diluted with the contents of the stomach. Gentian yellow prepares the stomach for digestion by increasing gastric secretions and the swelling of the mucous membranes. It accelerates the rate of absorption and elimination. This effect on the stomach occurs only three to eight minutes after ingestion. For these reasons, Europeans have concocted an "aperitif" out of gentian yellow, called "Suze," which originates from the south of France. It has since been adopted by North Americans as a good drink to increase the appetite. Gentian yellow helps absorb nutrients from food when it dilates the mucous membranes of the intestine about 20 to 35 minutes after it has been ingested. It also helps prevent fermentation of the food in the intestine.

Natural formulas to improve digestion or to enhance appetite usually contain a combination of extracts with high concentrations of bitters like the ones discussed. They are usually in the form of liquids but may also occur in tablet form. Although natural remedies are considered safe by the health industry, it is recommended that you consult a physician for digestive difficulties, since digestive disturbances are often associated with more serious illnesses.

Kidney Remedies

The kidneys filter toxins from our bodies, and these toxins are then removed via the urine. There are herbal remedies designed to clear the kidneys by promoting this effect. Essential oil of juniper promotes kidney filtration and is considered a diuretic.

Goldenrod *(Solidago virga aurea)* extract is a potent diuretic and helps remove toxins.

Extract of birch *(Betula alba)*, an antiseptic, is also a blood purifier, since it promotes the filtration of toxins. Knotweed *(Polygonum aviculare)* herbal extract also stimulates kidney function. Restharow *(Ononis spinosa)* extract is unique in increasing the volume of urine without overstressing the kidneys. Thus, although it regulates kidney function, the wrong dosage may induce the opposite effect.

A good herbal kidney remedy should contain an adjuvant

herb to help remineralize the system, because when a diuretic is used, even a natural one, precious minerals are lost. Including a herb such as horsetail *(Equisetum arvense)* will act as a remineralizing substance.

Most natural kidney remedies contain a combination of plant extracts that stimulate the kidneys, like the ones mentioned. These formulas generally occur as liquids. Although natural kidney remedies are deemed safe by the health industry, it is recommended that you consult a physician if you are bothered by symptoms such as difficulty in urinating, pain in the lower abdomen, blood-tinged urine, or incontinence, which are often associated with kidney ailments, before taking any kidney remedies, either natural or over-the-counter allopathic drugs.

Pain Remedies

This section describes commonly found extracts that relieve different kinds of pain.

Butterbur *(Petasites hybridus)* extract has been used for centuries all over Europe as an antispasmodic and to calm the nervous system processes that are related to pain in muscles and joints, as well as for stomach spasms. It is an alternative to allopathic analgesics, with the added benefit that it does not cause stomach acidity.

Willow *(Salix alba)* bark, has long been reputed for its antirheumatic properties. Studies in 1972 demonstrated that the glycoside salicyl alcohol in willow bark is changed in our bodies to salicylic acid. Salicylic acid reduces fever and relieves pain caused by swollen nerves and inflammation throughout the body.

The amino acid tryptophan, contained in meats and milk, has been found to significantly reduce the pain of root-canal therapy. According to researchers, tryptophan is converted to serotonin, a natural pain killer, in the body.

Just as there are foods that make you feel better when you

are sick, there are others that may aggravate certain conditions. For instance, *with migraines you should avoid vaso-active foods because migraine pain is due to the swelling of blood vessels. Some foods to avoid are cheeses and other dairy products, beans, citrus fruit, nuts, pickled and preserved foods, foods that contain nitrites, grapes, onions, caffeine, chocolate, and preservatives like monosodium glutamate.*

Essential oil of Roman chamomile *(Chamaemelum nobilis)* taken internally can reduce the pain of migraines by helping to constrict blood vessels and can act as a mild sedative and antispasmodic.

These are some of the more commonly available pain remedies that you can find at health food stores. Although they are deemed safe by the health industry, it is recommended that you also consult a physician when you experience pain.

Preventive Heart Remedies

There are several natural substances that act on the heart muscle. However, they should be viewed only as alternative medicines to be used under the guidance of a naturopath or holistic practitioner *after* medical diagnosis and treatment of a cardiac condition.

The best-known heart-related botanical is hawthorn *(Crataegus oxyacantha)*. Hawthorn contains flavonoids, which enlarge the coronary vessels, increasing the flow of blood to the heart. When the blood flow to the heart is increased, the heart muscle gets more oxygen, alleviating coronary stress.

Horse chestnut *(Aesculus hippocastanum)* extract is often used to increase circulation. This herb contains aescin, a vasodilator, which increases the flow of blood and the amount of oxygen delivered to the organs.

The condition of the blood plays an important role in the health of the heart. When the blood clots too rapidly, there is a higher risk of heart attack. Furthermore, a clot may become dislodged and flow to the heart, where blockage will occur. Blockage will injure the heart by cutting off the oxygen supply to the heart muscle. A clot is formed either by platelet aggregation or by the production of the blood protein fibrin.

Many natural remedies prevent platelet aggregation (formation of blood clots) Others stimulate the body's natural ability to dissolve clots. Garlic is the best-known blood-thinning substance. According to Dr. E. Block, chairman of the Department of Chemistry at the State University of New York, garlic contains ajoene, which interferes with the platelets' ability to stick together. Dr. Block suggests that ajoene may also inhibit the production of thromboxane, the chemical that causes clumping. Thus, garlic both dissolves clots and prevents clots from forming.

Vitamin E helps thin blood and prevents platelets from adhering to blood vessel walls. It protects blood vessels by maintaining their ability to manufacture prostacyclin, a naturally occurring chemical that prevents platelets from sticking to blood vessels and causing them injury.

Antioxidants other than vitamin E play an equally important role in cardiac health. Recent research suggests that damage occurs to the walls of blood vessels by free radical reactions and that this damage is a forerunner of cholesterol deposits. In fact, without this injury to the blood vessels, the cholesterol could not adhere to the walls of the vessels. Thus, antioxidants, which are free radical scavengers, can prevent the initial injury that leads to greater problems.

A 1982 study reported in the medical journal *Lancet* found that *the antioxidant selenium plays a significant role in preventing cardiovascular disease.*

Natural Remedies for Varicose Veins

Herring, tuna, wheat germ and bran, whole grains and yeast are selenium-rich foods. Selenium is available at health food stores as a micronutrient supplement, usually in the form of a tablet or a capsule. It may also be sold in the form of selenium-enriched yeast, which is not recommended, since manufacturers do not provide an estimate of the amount of selenium the yeast contains.

Varicose veins appear as a result of faulty blood vessel valves. For example, veins in our legs help transport blood from our legs back to our heart and lungs. As blood moves up the leg, the valves shut to prevent it from seeping backward. If these valves are too weak to prevent seepage, blood will collect in the vein, stretching its wall out of shape and forming a varicose vein. Some doctors recommend bioflavonoids from tangerines and oranges. Bioflavonoids strengthen the walls of veins, prevent dilation, and promote proper functioning of the valves.

Natural Blood Pressure Remedies

In several studies, the following nutrients were found to have a positive effect on blood pressure: magnesium, calcium, potassium, phosphorus, fiber, vegetable protein, starch, vitamin C, and vitamin D. Magnesium showed the greatest benefits. *Those who supplemented their diet with magnesium had significantly lower blood pressure.*

Natural Remedies for Healthy Eyes

A few innovative ophthalmologists are using nutritional therapy to treat serious eye conditions. Dr. G. P. Todd, 1985 author of *Nutrition, Health, and Disease,* is a leading authority on nutritional therapy for ophthalmic conditions. He reports using a multivitamin high in zinc to treat cataracts, with the remarkable result that they disappeared. Animal researchers have also shown that zinc deficiencies promoted cataracts.

Dr. Todd also uses nutritional therapy to treat glaucoma, a leading cause of blindness in adults. He has found that supplementing the diets of his glaucoma patients with manganese and vitamin A reverses the condition, to the point where about 40 percent of his patients can stop using prescription eye drops and remain on only nutritional therapy.

Subsequent investigation by Dr. S. P. Varna into the cause of cataracts revealed that the lens of the eye is damaged by free radicals. Because free radicals are the product of oxidation reactions, and tissue in the eye is particularly prone to oxidation, since light promotes damaging oxidation reactions, the result is that the lens loses its transparency. Thus, antioxidants can offset this damage by scavenging the free radicals, and ophthalmologists have been able to improve many conditions in their patients. For instance, Dr. Varna, an ophthalmologist at the University of Maryland Medical School, now prescribes vitamins C and E, after he and his colleagues found that these nutrients protected lenses exposed to free radicals.

After years of opthalmological research, Dr. E. J. Crary found that nutritional therapy reversed two serious eye diseases: diabetic retinopathy and senile macular degeneration. Diabetic retinopathy is a disease of the retina. Dr. Crary believes that there is a buildup of free radicals in the blood vessels of the diseased eyes and has used antioxidants to treat them, with a 70 percent reduction in overall disease. In 90 percent of patients with senile macular degeneration, Dr. Crary has reported complete reversal and restoration of vision.

Other researchers have found that vitamin E prevents a disease of the retina leading to blindness, caused by oxygen therapy in premature or low-birth-weight infants.

Autoimmune Diseases and Natural Remedies

An autoimmune disease is one in which the immune system turns against the body. Instead of destroying invaders, the components of our immune system invade the cells of the tissues and fluids of our bodies. In rheumatoid arthritis, for example, the immune system's defense cells attack the joints' soft tissue and fluids. This process releases free radicals, which further damage surrounding connective tissue and attract more defense cells to invade the site. This causes tissue inflammation, and a painful cycle commences.

Because autoimmune diseases generate free radicals, it follows that antioxidants can be helpful in controlling such diseases. Studies have conclusively shown that vitamin A and vitamin E decrease free-radical-induced inflammation. *A German study has found vitamin E to be the leading remedy to treat arthritic inflammation.* Other studies have shown that copper can also reduce arthritic inflammation by scavenging superoxide and hydrogen peroxide, two oxygen radicals. Copper, zinc, and manganese are components of super oxide dismutase (SOD), the enzyme found in all cells that detoxifies free radicals. There are commercial products that describe themselves as SOD, but studies have shown that consuming SOD does not promote the natural formation of SOD in the body. In fact, SOD consumed orally is inactivated by the gastrointestinal tract and thus has no value. Other studies reveal that the intravenous injection of SOD has little value, since SOD survives for only a short period of time in the bloodstream. Since copper, zinc, and manganese are components that naturally form SOD, consuming these nutrients orally will contribute to the production of SOD in the body.

Autoimmune disease may attack the soft tissue and the fluid in joints, causing the inflammation and pain common to such diseases as rheumatoid arthritis. A physician specializing in rheumatoid conditions should be consulted. Many of these doctors are holistic practitioners who will recommend vitamin therapy.

Cancer and Natural Remedies

Cancer is a collective term that encompasses many diseases characterized by unruly cellular division. There are two phases to cancer: initiation and promotion. Initiation occurs when a cancer-causing substance damages the genetic material of the cell, inducing mutation. Unlike initiation, promotion is reversible; that is, when the promoter is removed, the damaging process stops.

It is the initiators that are insidiously dangerous. *Often the lapse between initiation and the appearance of a tumor is 10 years or more, and diagnosis by the appearance of a recognizable tumor may come too late.* Moreover, there are two types of initiators: direct carcinogens and procarcinogens. These are either agents that enter the body in their active form, or those that must be transformed into their proximate form (their ultimately active chemical form). For example, nitrites (see chapter 9) form nitrosamines, which is the cancer-causing compound (proximate form) of nitrites and nitrates. Thus nitrites from processed meats or nitrates in vegetables must be activated to form their proximate or carcinogenic form, nitrosamine. But a stimulus like radiation will directly cause DNA damage, beginning the insidious process of cancer.

Unfortunately, free radicals are major factors in activating procarcinogens. Worse is the fact that certain carcinogens like nitrosamines generate oxidants. Studies have shown that cancerous tissue contains a high level of oxidants and that these oxidants are in turn initiators and promoters of cancer.

The use of natural remedies in the fight against cancer has come a long way in the last decade. The most revealing proof of this is the research in this field supported by the National Cancer Institute. Approximately 30 clinical trials in cancer prevention have been under way since 1983 (see page 196). Current studies have revealed that the cancer mechanism can indeed be inhibited by nutrients, at the initiation phase, by boosting the immune system to delay the growth of tumors.

Vitamin A

Studies have produced irrefutable evidence that certain vitamins not only prevent cancer but can be used to treat certain types of cancer. Vitamin A is probably the most significant. A 1973 study at the National Cancer Institute revealed that vitamin A was effective against cancer of the colon. Another study found that vitamin A supplemented in the diet significantly reduced lung cancer. In clinical studies on cancer patients, vitamin A was found to significantly reduce carcinomas, and topically applied vitamin A reduced malignant melanomas.

Because vitamin A is an antioxidant, it scavenges free radicals. But according to researchers, this is not the main anticancer function of vitamin A. The main action of vitamin A is to activate the immune system. A clinical study has demonstrated that T-cells were greatly increased in lung cancer patients—a factor that helped to prolong life.

Vitamin C

Certainly the best-known study of vitamin C as a treatment for cancer is the study done by Nobel Prize winner and eminent scientist Linus Pauling and E. Cameron. In this study, vitamin C was supplemented to terminal cancer patients. The results were reported to increase the length of life of the vitamin-treated group five times that of the untreated control group.

Recent studies have shown that vitamin C decreases the harmful effect of carcinogens by altering them chemically so that they can be excreted by the body. It also stimulates T-cell function, decreases the immune-suppressant hormones, and raises blood levels of interferon, our natural antibiotic. Pauling reported that vitamin C protected against nitrite initiators by preventing nitrite from forming into carcinogenic nitrosamine.

Many other studies have shown that vitamin C is effective in exerting protection against malignant stomach, colon, esophagus, and bladder tumors, and protects us against certain carcinogens, viruses, and radiation.

Vitamin E

Epidemiologic studies have revealed that the more vitamin E you con-

sume, the less are your chances of getting cancer. Studies into the effects of vitamin E on immunity reveal that vitamin E increases T-cell activity, as well as other factors of the immune system, such as antibody responses to antigens. Still other studies have shown that vitamin E decreases the production of prostaglandin that is a known immunosuppressant.

Like vitamin C, vitamin E also works to inhibit damaging reactions caused by nitrites and amines.

Selenium

Over 60 studies have indicated that the trace mineral selenium may be beneficial in the prevention of cancer.

It is important to note, though, that selenium as a trace mineral is toxic at high levels. Unlike vitamins that are often supplemented for therapy at dosages 100 times the recommended dietary allowance, minerals should not be consumed, even therapeutically, in dosages exceeding 3 times the RDA values.

Selenium is known to inhibit epithelial-type tumors such as those of the stomach, colon, lung, liver, kidney, oral cavity, mammary glands, and skin. Selenium has also been shown to reduce tumors due to radiation and viruses and to protect against heavy metal toxicity from mercury, lead, and cadmium. It is also a potent immune stimulant.

There is an important difference between organic and synthetic selenium. Some animal studies have shown that the synthetic form, sodium selenite, is more effective than selenocysteine, the natural form, in preventing cancer. Other studies report that there is no difference between the effects of organic and synthetic selenium. However, to date most of the related research has been done using synthetic selenium.

Selenium is even more valuable when combined with vitamin E and with such other antioxidants as glutathione. One 1988 study found that moderate intake of selenium combined with high levels of vitamin E reduced mammary tumors in animals and suggests that the combination is a feasible chemopreventive therapy for cancer protection in humans. A 1987 Japanese study suggested a link between low selenium blood levels and the incidence of lung cancer in humans.

Calcium

Clinical trials in 1986 supported by the National Cancer Institute, and a 1985 study published in the *New England Journal of Medicine,* suggest that dietary calcium significantly reduces abnormal cells in patients with high risk for colon cancer and that it is beneficial in reversing precancerous conditions.

Bioflavonoids

Bioflavonoids are organic compounds found in plants. To date, nearly 1,000 compounds have been isolated. Bioflavonoids are sometimes referred to as vitamins. *A number of studies have shown that bioflavonoids inhibit the initiation and promotion phases of cancer.* Bioflavonoids appear to prevent the invasion of tumors into healthy tissue by stabilizing collagen, the protein found in healthy connective tissue.

Essential Oils

Recently, essential oil of orange and other citrus fruits have received much attention in relation to cancer. Their anticancerous component is a terpene, limonene. According to one leading researcher, limonene taken internally is able to lower the incidence of cancers caused by chemical carcinogens. Although terpenic essential oils can be safely consumed in minute quantities, an aromatherapist should be consulted before you take any essential oils (see chapter 6).

Studies of essential oil of garlic have also reported that components of garlic may result in complete inhibition of cancers caused by nitrosamines. One animal study found garlic more effective than conventional immunotherapy in reducing bladder tumors in animals.

Coenzyme Q_{10}

The study of coenzyme Q_{10} (CoQ_{10}) and cancer began when a 1968 study showed that cancerous tissue was deficient in Q_{10}. One chemotherapy cancer study noted a deficiency in patients with advanced cancer. As an antioxidant, CoQ_{10} can be expected to have a protective effect against cancer by intervening in the vicious biochemical cycle of free radical damage. It enhances macrophage functions and increases antibody activity. Furthermore, it has shown antimicrobial activity against such pathogens as fungi, bacteria, and even viruses.

The current findings relating natural remedies to specific ailments provide scientific evidence on the therapeutic properties of these substances. However, the above information should not be used for self-diagnosis or self-medication. Holistic practitioners should be consulted for specific diagnosis, medications, and dosages of all natural remedies.

FOR FURTHER READING

Balansky, R., and Agirova, R. "Sodium Selenite Inhibition of the Reproduction of Some Oncogenic RNA-Viruses." *Experientia* 37 (1981).

Bauer, R. et al. "Immunological in Vivo Examinations of Echinacea Extracts." *Arzneim-Forsch* 38 (1988).

Beisel, W. "Single Nutrients and Immunity." *American Journal of Clinical Nutrition* 35 (1982).

Beisel, W. R.; Edelman, R.; Nauss, K.; and Suskind, R. M. "Single Nutrient Effects on Immunologic Functions." *Journal of the American Medical Association* 245 (1981).

Belman, S. "Onion and Garlic Oils Inhibit Tumor Promotion." *Carcinogenesis* 4 (1983).

Bistrian, B., Blackburn, G. L.; Scrimshaw, N. S.; Flatt, J. P. "Cellular Immunity in Semi-starved States in Hospitalized Adults." *American Journal of Clinical Nutrition* 28 (October 1975).

Bistrian, B., Blackburn, G., Hallowell, E., Heddle, R. "Protein Statis of General Surgical Patients." *Journal of the American Medical Association* 230 (November 11, 1974).

Blankenhorn, Gunter. "Vitamin E—New Results from Clinical Research in Europe." *VERIS Vitamin E* (Spring 1986).

Block, E. et al. "Ajoene: A Potent Antithrombotic Agent from Garlic." *Journal of the American Chemical Society* 106 (1984).

Cameron, E., and Pauling, L. "Ascorbic Acid As a Therapeutic Agent in Cancer." *Journal of the International Academy of Preventive Medicine* 5 (1979).

Cameron, E., and Pauling, L. "Supplemental Ascorbate in the Supportive Treatment of Cancer: Prolongation of Survival Times in Terminal Human Cancer." *Proceedings of the National Academy of Sciences, USA* 73 (1976).

Cerklewski, E., and Forbes, R. "Influence of Dietary Selenium on Lead Toxicity in the Rat." *Journal of Nutrition* 106 (1976).

Cerutti, P. "Prooxidant States and Tumor Promotion." *Science* 227 (1985).

Cross, C. et al. "Oxygen Radicals and Human Disease." *Annals of Internal Medicine* 107 (1987).

Dewys, W. et al. "Clinical Trials in Cancer Prevention." *Cancer* 58 (1986).

Dörling, Eberhard. "Bio-Strath R (Plasmolysed Yeast Solution) and Increased Performance: A Double Blind Trial of Bio-Strath on 60 Subjects." *Swiss Pharma* 3 (1981).

Duchateau, J.; Delepesse, G.; and Vereecke, P. "Influence of Oral Zinc Supplementation on the Lymphocyte Response to Mitogens of Normal Subjects." *American Journal of Clinical Nutrition* 34 (1987).

Duchateau, J.; Delepesse, G.; Vrijens, R.; and Collet, H. "Beneficial Effects of Oral Zinc Supplementation on the Immune Response of Old People." *American Journal of Medicine* 70 (1981).

Elson, C. et al. "Anti-carcinogenic Activity of D-Limonene during the Initiation and Promotion/Progression Stages of DMBA-induced Rat Mammary Carcinogenesis." *Carcinogenesis* 9 (1988).

Facinelli, Paul. "A Repair Kit for Varicose Veins." *Prevention* (March 1985).

Fraker, P. J. et al. "Regeneration of T-cell Helper Function in Zinc-deficient Adult Mice." *Proceedings of the National Academy of Sciences, USA* 75 (1978).

Fritz-Niggli, Hedi, and Michel, C. "Effects of a Yeast Preparation on Radiation induced Developmental Anomalies." *Swiss Med* 5 (1983).

Grobbee, D., and Hofman, A. "Effect of Calcium Supplementation on Diastolic Blood Pressure in Young People with Mild Hypertension." *Lancet* 2 (1986).

Hufnagel, V. *No More Hysterectomies.* New York: New American Library, 1988.

Ip, C., "Feasibility of Using Lower Doses of Chemopreventive Agents in a Combination Regimen for Cancer Protection." *Cancer Letters* 39 (1988).

Joffres, M. et al. "Relationship of Magnesium Intake and Other Dietary Factors to Blood Pressure: The Honolulu Heart Study." *American Journal of Clinical Nutrition* 45 (1987).

Karanja, N.; Morris, C.; Illingworth, D.; and McCarron, D. "Plasma Lipids and Hypertension: Response to Calcium Supplementation." *American Journal of Clinical Nutrition* 45 (1987).

Khaw, K., and Barrett-Connor, E. "Dietary Potassium and Stroke-associated Mortality." *New England Journal of Medicine* 316 (1987).

Kraemer, K. et. al "Prevention of Skin Cancer in Xerodema Pigmentosum with the Use of Oral Isoretinoin." *New England Journal of Medicine* 318 (1988).

Leibovitz, B. "Selenium: The Misunderstood Mineral." *Nutrition Update* 4 (1986).

Leslie, G. B. "Effect of Bio-Strath R (Plasmolysed Yeast Solution) Treatment on the Duration and Recovery from an Anaesthetic Dose of Hexobarbitone Sodium in Mice." *Swiss Med* 4 (1985).

Leslie, G. B. "A Pharmacometric Evaluation of Nine Bio-Strath Herbal Remedies." *Medita* 8 (1978).

Lipkin, M., and Newmark, H. "Effect of Added Dietary Calcium on Colonic Epithelial-Cell Proliferation in Subjects at High Risk for Colonic Cancer." *New England Journal of Medicine* 313 (1985).

Lorenzi, G., and Cogoli, A. "Effect of Plasmolysed Yeast Preparations on Cellular Functions." *Swiss Biotech* 3 (1985).

Machlin, L. J., and Bendich, A. "Free Radical Tissue Damage: Protective Role of Antioxidant Nutrients." *Federation of American Societies for Experimental Biology Journal* 1 (1987).

Maleskey, G. "Thin Your blood and Live Longer." *Prevention* (May 1987).

Maltzman, T.; Tanner, M.; Elson, C.; and Gould, M. "Anticarcinogenic Activity of Specific Orange Peel Oil Monoterpenes." *Federation Proceedings* 45 (1986).

Marnett, L. "Peroy Free Radicals: Potential Mediators of Tumor Initiation and Promotion." *Carcinogenesis* 8 (1987).

Marsh, C. et al. "Superiority of Intravesical Immunotherapy with *Corynebacterium Parvum* and *Allium Sativum* in Control of Murine Bladder Cancer. *Journal of Urology* 137 (1987).

Mayer, F., and Menge, F., *Arzt u. Patient* 62 (1949).

McCormick, D.; Burns, F.; and Albert, R. "Inhibition of Rat Mammary Carcinogenesis by Short Dietary exposure to Retinyl Acetate." *Cancer Research* 20 (1967).

Medina, D., and Morrison, D. "Current Ideas on Selenium As a Chemopreventive Agent." *Pathological and Immunopathological Research* 7 (1988).

Meydani, S. et al. "Vitamin E Supplementation Suppresses Prostaglandin E_2 Synthesis and Enhances the Immune Response of Aged Mice." *Mechanisms of Aging and Development* 34 (1986).

Michel, C., and Fritz-Niggli, Hedi. "Effects of a Yeast Preparation and Low Dosage Irradiation on Fertility in White Mice." *Radiologia Clinica et Biologica (Internation Radiologica Review)*, no. 3 (1973).

Micksche, M. et al. "Stimulation of Immune Response in Lung Cancer Patients by Vitamin A Therapy." *Oncology* 34 (1977).

Miyamoto, H., et al. "Serum Selenium and Vitamin E concentrations in Families of Lung Cancer Patients." *Cancer* 60 (1987).

Perchellet, J.; Perchellet, E.; Abney, N.; Zirnstein, J.; and Belman, S. "Effects of Garlic and Onion Oils on Glutathione Peroxidase Activity, the Ratio of Reduced/Oxidized Glutathione and Ornithine Decarboxylase Induction in Isolated Mouse Epidermal Cells Treated with Tumor Promoters." *Cancer Biochemistry and Biophysics* 8 (1986).

Phillips, M., and Baetz, A., ed. *Diet and Resistance to Disease.* New York: Plenum Press, 1981.

Poirier, K., and Milner, J. "Factors Influencing the Antitumorigenic Properties of Selenium in Mice." *Journal of Nutrition* 113 (1983).

Salonen, J. T. et al. "Association between Cardiovascular Death and Myocardial Infarction and Serum Selenium in a Matched-Pair Longitudinal Study." *Lancet* 2 (1982).

Serrentino, Jo, *Herbal Remedies: Therapeutic Use.* Technical manual. Montreal: Bioforce, 1989.

Sharma, V. et al. "Antibacterial Property of Allium Sativum Linn: In Vivo and in Vitro Studies." *Indian Journal of Experimental Biology* 15 (1977).

Shichiri, M. et al. "Apparent Low Levels of Ubiquinone in Rat and Human Neoplastic Tissues." *International Journal for Vitamin and Nutrition Research* 38 (1968).

Sinha, S. et al. "Vitamin E Supplementation Reduces Frequency of Periventricular Hemorrhage in Very Preterm Babies." *Lancet* 1 (1987).

Staff. "Tryptophan Takes the Bite Out of Pain." *Prevention* (July 1985).

Sugawara, N., and Sugawara, C. "Selenium Protection against Testicular Lipid Peroxidation from Cadmium." *Journal of Applied Biochemistry* 6 (1984).

Sumino, K.; Yamamoto, R.; and Kitamura, S. A. "Role of Selenium against Methylmercury Toxicity." *Nature* 268 (1977).

Varma, S. D.; Kumar S.; Richards, R. D. "Light-induced Damage to Ocular Lens Cation-pump: Prevention by Vitamin C." *Proceedings of the National Academy of Sciences* (July 1979).

Vogel, A. *Le Petit Docteur.* Teufen, Switzerland: HAR, 1978.

Wagner, H.; Zenk, M. H.; and Ott, H. "Polysaccharides Derived from Echinacea Plants as Immunostimulants." *Patent-Ger Offen* 3 (1988).

Watson, R. "Immunological Enhancement by Fat-soluble Vitamins, Minerals, and Trace Metals: A Factor in Cancer Prevention." *Cancer Detection and Prevention* 9 (1986).

Weiner, M. A. *Earth Medicine.* New York: Macmillan, 1980.

Will, Andrew. *Natural Health, Natural Medicine.* Boston: Houghton-Mifflin, 1990.

Zarrow, Susan. "Keep Your Eyes Young and Sharp." *Prevention* (March 1985).

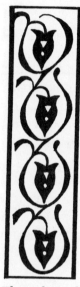

THIRTEEN

Commonly Asked Questions about Natural Remedies

1. *Can you still take vitamin C if you are prone to kidney problems?*

There have been cases where vitamin C supplements have provoked kidney stones in both people and animals. This happens because vitamin C may sometimes cause oxalic acid to accumulate. The amount of this acid produced in your body depends on the foods you eat. For instance, a diet high in meats produces a large amount of oxalic acid, which then settles in the kidneys in the form of kidney stones. Warning signs of oxalic acid buildup, before kidney stones form, include sore joints and rheumatic-type pain, a pungent body odor, and skin conditions such as eczema.

However, those prone to kidney stones can still take vitamin C supplements, if they take them with vitamin B_6. Vitamin B_6 helps rid the body of oxalic acid, thereby neutralizing the harmful effects of ascorbic acid. Usually equal amounts of vitamin C and vitamin B_6 should be taken, but it is always best to consult an expert for the exact concentrations of supplements that you require.

2. *Do chewable vitamin C tablets corrode your teeth?*

Studies have shown that the acidity level of chewable ascorbic acid tablets can irreversibly damage the pearly-white enamel on our teeth. The corrosive acid gradually eats away at enamel and even fillings, causing calcium loss in teeth.

The solution is to take a chewable vitamin C tablet that binds ascorbic acid to calcium. This is known as calcium ascorbate, and unlike pure ascorbic acid, it is nonacidic. Vitamin C tablets made of calcium ascorbate are also gentler on the stomach, as they do not promote stomach acidity. Moreover, they provide a sound source of calcium.

Watch out for the sugar content in chewable ascorbic acid tablets as well. Make sure they are sweetened with pure fruit juices or fructose and not sugar, which causes the release of a large amount of insulin, leading to fluctuating blood sugar and hunger pangs. Sugar also promotes cavities.

3. *Why do you lose weight when you are ill? Is there anything you can do about it?*

You lose weight when you are ill because amino acid deficiency causes muscles to waste. Under stress, pain, anxiety, infection, and viruses, amino acids within the body are converted by the liver to glucose, a blood sugar. This makes you lose nitrogen from muscle protein because amino acids are being taken from tissues. The amino acid deficiencies become a vicious circle as they steadily deplete the fundamental elements of the body, reducing your resistance and greatly taxing the immune system. In this sense, you can literally waste away.

All this can be prevented by supplementing with amino acids. You can take a complete amino acid supplement, one that contains all of the amino acids, or a food substance that contains amino acids, like yeast or chlorella. Remember to choose pancreatic digests of protein (see chapter 9) if you take amino acid complexes, and if you are taking yeast, a plasmolyzed yeast solution.

4. *What is provitamin A or beta carotene?*

Provitamin A is a nontoxic form of vitamin A, also known as the precursor of vitamin A. Vitamin A from animal sources (fish oils) is a retinoid, whereas provitamin A is from plant sources and is a carotenoid. Provitamin A is most commonly known as beta carotene, but alpha and gamma carotene are also sold as provitamin A.

The main properties of beta carotene are its antioxidant effect and the neutralizing of free radical reactions. Research has also shown that beta carotene is effective against malignant tumors.

You can find beta carotene in dry or oil form. It is water soluble and measured in international units (IU). It is more stable in its dry form.

5. *What do* EPA *and* DHA *on product labels stand for?*

These letters stand for fatty acids found in marine fish oils. EPA stands for eicosapentenoic acid, and DHA stands for docosahexenoic acid. They are both polyunsaturated fats and come mainly from deep, cold-water marine fish, mainly salmon, herring, bluefish, and mackerel, and certain shellfish, like crab. These fish feed on marine chlorella, which contains these fats.

These fish oils have been found to prevent and successfully treat heart disease by improving the type of lipoproteins in the blood—reducing the low-density lipoprotein (LDL) and very low density lipoprotein (VLDL) cholesterol while increasing high-density lipoprotein (HDL) cholesterol. Fish oils also prevent blood clotting by increasing the production of a hormone that blocks the clotting action.

Still more, *marine fish oils have anti-inflammatory effects.* They prevent the release of such substances as histamine and leukotrienes, which cause inflammation. A 1985 article in *Lancet* reported successful treatment of rheumatoid arthritis with fish oils.

Although all of these benefits point to the virtues of marine fish oils, there is one serious drawback with commercial omega-

3 fish oils. Because they are highly unsaturated, they are unstable and susceptible to damage by oxygen, leading to free radicals in tissues and to disease. So fish oils should be supplemented with such antioxidants as vitamin E, selenium, and fat-soluble vitamin C. They should be packaged in nitrogen-flushed containers (containers free of air). Look for fish oils supplemented with vitamin E and ascorbyl palmitate (fat-soluble vitamin C).

Studies indicate that EPA and DHA are nontoxic and do not produce side effects. However, because of their anticlotting capacity, persons with bleeding disorders such as hemophelia should not take fish oils or should consult a physician before doing so.

6. *What can I do to lower my blood cholesterol?*
Exercise, diet, and supplements can change your serum cholesterol level. What you eat is probably the most important factor. Believe it or not, cutting down on saturated fats is more important than cutting down on cholesterol.

Supplementing your diet with fiber helps to lower cholesterol. Forty to 60 grams of fiber a day will help bind cholesterol to bile salts so that it can be eliminated from the body. Researchers at the Veterans Administration Medical Center in Kentucky found that a high-fiber diet decreased LDL by 23 percent and total serum cholesterol levels by 19 percent.

Niacin has been found to lower the level of "bad" cholesterol, LDL, while increasing "good" cholesterol, HDL. It is medically recognized as a cholesterol fighter and is listed as such in the *Physician's Desk Reference* (under its chemical name *nicotinic acid*).

Vitamin C is another recognized cholesterol fighter. Many scientific studies have shown that taking vitamin C results in a decreased level of serum cholesterol. Citrus essential oils are usually used holistically as therapy for reducing cholesterol rather than preventing it.

Lecithin is also a good cholesterol fighter because, as a natural emulsifier, it binds with fats to carry them out of the body. It also increases HDL while decreasing LDL.

Sitosterol is considered a cholesterol neutralizer. Derived from plants, it is white and waxy, resembling cholesterol. One researcher claims that if you consume sitosterol along with cholesterol-laden foods, you need not worry about the cholesterol.

Sitosterol is plentiful in corn oil but is destroyed by heat during processing. So use cold-pressed natural corn oil, or extra virgin corn oil. Sitosterol supplements are scarce, but they are available in some parts of the United States and are becoming more widely available.

Garlic and onion extracts stimulate production of HDL while reducing LDL.

To fight cholesterol, 500 milligrams of niacin per day is usually required, and between 700 milligrams and 1 gram of vitamin C. But as in all questions of nutrition and supplementation, it is best to consult a professional for the appropriate dosages associated with your diet and lifestyle.

7. What's CoQ_{10}?

Coenzyme Q_{10} is a natural nutrient found in many foods and in human tissue. It is particularly abundant in the heart muscle and in the tissues of the gums. Coenzyme Q_{10} is involved in energy metabolism at the cellular level, and it has an effect on the total energy picture of the body and subsequently the functioning of organs, particularly the heart. CoQ_{10} actually increases the cardiac contractions without stressing the heart because it also lowers blood pressure. *Research has shown that in many cases of heart disease there has been a deficiency in the concentration of* CoQ_{10}.

CoQ_{10} given orally as tablets or by injection has been used in the treatment of congestive heart failure, arrhythmias (irregular heartbeat), and angina pectoris (heart pain). Periodontists have also been using it recently to treat gum disease.

8. *Should lecithin be taken as liquid, granules, or capsules?*
The form in which lecithin is taken is not that important. What
is important is the way it is processed. Lecithin granules are usually defatted, bleached, and or deodorized—processes that destroy phosphatidylcholine, the active ingredient of lecithin.
Look for an indication on the label that there is between 20 percent and 55 percent phosphatidylcholine in a lecithin product.
(The high concentration, 55 percent, of phosphatidylcholine is
very expensive.)

9. *Which natural remedies can boost the immune system?*
Many vitamins, as well as some plant extracts, act as immune
stimulants.

Such immune stimulants include the antioxidants zinc, vitamins A, E, and C, and the trace mineral selenium, the nutrient
glutathione, and the coenzyme Q_{10}.

The principal action of an immune booster is to stimulate the
activity of T-cells. These cells attack foreign cells by producing
antibodies. T-cells are directed by the thymus gland, and so a
good immune booster will also encourage proper thymus gland
functioning. Research has shown that the aforementioned nutrients stimulate T-cell activity and function.

Studies have shown that vitamin C stimulates effector cells,
which are a type of protective cell, and that it also protects effector cells from their free radical by-products.

Pantotheine, the coenzyme form of pantothenic acid (vitamin B_5), also stimulates T-cell activity.

Beta carotene deactivates free radicals.

Echinacea extract stimulates the formation of antibodies, inhibits hyaluronidase, responsible for spreading a virus throughout the body, and increases the production of interferon, involved in immunity.

Astragalus, often packaged as the Chinese herb *Qiang gan
ruan jian tang*, is known to stimulate the immune system. It acti-

vates T-cells, helps to produce interferon, and has been found to destroy viruses.

Garlic and onion contain many tumor-inhibiting substances, but it is the selenium within these allium vegetables that gives them antioxidant properties.

The tropical plant known as mathaké *(Terminalia spp)* is considered an immune enhancer.

White willow enhances the immune system by inhibiting the immune suppressant immunoglobulin PGE_2.

Certain mushrooms are gaining recognition as immune stimulants. Studies indicate that injection of reishi *(Ganoderma lucidum)* mushroom extract enhances the immune system. The shiitake mushroom contains lentinan, an ingredient that has been shown to kill viruses, to stimulate interferon, and to stimulate T-cell and other killer cell activity, as well as to prevent tumors. Lentinan has been used for years to treat cancer in Japan. Whether the consumption of fresh, reconstituted, or dehydrated mushrooms, or even the extract of these mushrooms, is beneficial is not yet known, since research was done with injections of specially prepared solutions.

Finally, experiments in Japan reveal the immune-enhancing effects of chlorella, which also has antiviral and antitumor effects and greatly stimulates the production of interferon.

Antioxidants are being identified every day, and there are many other immune stimulants. When you are reading about potential immune stimulants, it is important to look for conclusive research and not to rely on hearsay.

10. *I've heard about the toxicity of vitamin A. Is it dangerous to take vitamin A supplements?*

There has been much discussion about the safe dosages of vitamin A. The Recommended Dietary Allowances (RDA) have frightened consumers, and the government has not published the facts about vitamin A. In the first place, vitamin A or retinol is the form of vitamin A found in animal tissue. Carotene is the form of provitamin A found in plant tissue. The RDA claims that levels higher than 5000 IU of vitamin A may be toxic in human males, yet dosages of prepared vitamin A are between 10 000 and 25 000 IU (depending on the country the product is sold in). The controversy has arisen from the therapeutic use of vitamin A in the treatment and prevention of diseases such as cancer. Reactions that occur from long-term use of high doses of vitamin A may include dry skin, headaches, and fatigue, and have been observed clinically when doses of over 100 000 IU a day have been taken for approximately 13 months. But all symptoms disappeared following discontinuation of the supplement. Other studies have shown that it took 7½ months for symptoms of toxicity to develop after consumption of 300 000 IU a day. However, no toxic effects have been observed in people taking 50 000 IU a day over a long period of time. Thus, vitamin A shows no toxic side effects at levels 10 times the RDA.

Although experts are still debating the optimum level of vitamin A, one 1976 study suggests that the "ideal" daily allowance of vitamin A is 33 000 IU. New studies on the benefits of vitamin A are appearing in the scientific literature every year, which no doubt will alter the "ideal" daily allowance of vitamin A.

If you are still worried about taking vitamin A but want a supplement, take beta carotene, the nontoxic vitamin A precursor, also known as provitamin A.

11. What are medium-chain triglycerides?

Medium-chain triglycerides (MTC) are found as supplements in health food stores. Misunderstanding of these useful lipids stems from their name, triglycerides, which makes everyone think of cholesterol. In fact, medium-chain triglycerides are used as a source of energy. They are resistant to rancidity, are easily absorbed and metabolized by the body, and contain twice the energy of carbohydrates. Since 1950, North American hospitals have used MTCS to boost energy in recovering patients. MTCS have been shown to reduce body fat, lower cholesterol, and improve the metabolism of carbohydrates and proteins, as well as increase the absorption of minerals. Recent investigation of the use of MCTS in reversing obesity is encouraging. MTCS are mostly commonly used by athletes or body builders to increase energy for performance and to decrease recovery time after a hard workout.

12. *What is* CSA?

CSA stands for the nutrient chondroitin sulphate A. Research has revealed that substantial levels of CSA occur naturally in the aorta—the largest blood vessel that leads to the heart. CSA is responsible for the health of the circulatory system because the viscosity, permeability, ion exchange, and other processes that occur within the cells and intercellular matrix of the arterial walls depend on CSA levels. Unfortunately, as we age, natural CSA levels diminish. *When the CSA levels are reduced, the bloodstream and the aorta become vulnerable to attack, mostly by cholesterol-containing plaque deposits.*

In a Japanese medical study, CSA was used to treat high levels of blood fats. Results showed that CSA was responsible for clearing cholesterol from human aorta.

CSA is also an anticoagulant. Research has shown conclusively that CSA can dissolve clots just as well as widely used drugs like heparin and dicumoral but without any of their dangerous side effects.

CSA is also anti-inflammatory, antiallergic, and antistress. Clinical observation has found that CSA is successful in treating and preventing osteoporosis and in accelerating the healing of bone fractures. So successful are treatments with CSA that rheumatologist physicians are using topical applications of CSA for inflammatory connective tissue diseases. After 20 years of medical use, there are no confirmed reports of CSA toxicity. In addition, more than 20,000 patients in Japan are treated every day with CSA (on the average, 10 grams daily for a 6-year period), without any evidence of toxic effects.

However, as with all natural remedies, the way CSA is manufactured is of the utmost importance. *CSA products must contain 100 percent CSA extracted from calf trachea.* Moreover, these extracts must be purified, for allergies often result from contaminated extracts or from extracts containing residues. Desiccated (dehydrated) extracts are not the same and should be avoided. Likewise, beware of CSA products made from dehydrated seaweed or Irish moss, which contain only traces of CSA. An additional proof of purity when buying a CSA product is the analysis or the guarantee of 100 percent purified bovine CSA extract from an independent laboratory (a laboratory other than that of the manufacturer).

You may see glandulars marketed as CSA, but they are not the same substance. Glandulars are polypeptides and nucleopeptides, whereas CSA is a mucopolysaccharide, a complex protein. Moreover, glandulars are extremely unstable in the digestive tract. CSA has been tested for digestive stability and found to be extremely stable, remaining unchanged in the urine.

13. *What is the value of octacosanol in wheat germ oil?*
Octacosanol is a long-chain fatty alcohol derived from wheat germ oil and is responsible for many of the benefits of wheat germ oil. Most wheat germ oil, however, only contains about 0.01 to 0.005 percent octacosanol. It is thought to prevent miscarriage. Pioneer research with octacosanol has shown that it improves strength, stamina, and muscle reaction time. Another study revealed that *octacosanol can stimulate the repair of damaged neurons in the spinal cord and brain.* Further studies with damaged-neuron-related diseases like muscular sclerosis and amyotrophic lateral sclerosis have been extremely promising.

Octacosanol is an example of an extract where extraction seems warranted, as there is so little of the substance in pure wheat germ oil. To get a useful dose, a large amount of wheat germ oil would have to be consumed, meaning that a lot of polyunsaturated and saturated fats would be consumed also.

14. *Which is better, coffee or tea to wash down vitamins?*
Neither. Both contain forms of caffeine, and caffeine destroys or diminishes the action of many vitamins. Furthermore, chlorogenic acid, an ingredient in both caffeinated and decaffeinated coffee, destroys thiamine in the body.

15. *Does the gel straight from the aloe vera plant have the same properties as aloe extract?*
No, because the gel straight from the plant is not a stable substance. It may relieve the sting of a minor burn on contact, but it does not possess the medicinal properties of properly extracted aloe vera, which include antifungal, antibacterial, antibiotic, and regenerative properties. To capture these properties, a mature, four-year-old aloe vera plant must be used together with cold-press extraction.

16. *What is oil of evening primrose used for?*
As its name implies, oil of evening primrose is the natural oil extracted from the seed of the evening primrose, a wildflower. This oil is rich in gamma-linoleic acid (GLA), which leads to the production of prostaglandins, a group of essential fatty acids present in all tissues of the human body. Prostaglandins are essential to the proper functioning of all organs and of the reproductive system. Hundreds of well-documented studies of oil of evening primrose have revealed its beneficial effects in the treatment and prevention of cardiac and vascular conditions, arterial tension, rheumatoid arthritis, eczema, asthma, allergies, obesity, multiple sclerosis, hyperactivity, and premenstrual syndrome.

Oil of evening primrose has received most of its praise for its relief of premenstrual syndrome (PMS)—a condition that affects women before the onset of menstruation and that is characterized by uncomfortable physical and mental symptoms. The symptoms of PMS occur when there are low prostaglandin E_1 levels in the bloodstream, caused by the hormonal changes that occur before menstruation. Prostaglandin E_1 is manufactured from gamma-linoleic acid (GLA). Oil of evening primrose is a rich natural source of GLA and supplementation substantially increases prostaglandin E_1 levels, according to researchers who tested hundreds of women. This research, linking prostaglandin E_1 to PMS, received a Nobel Prize in 1982.

Beware, however, because not all oil of evening primrose products are created equal. Look for a product that has been analyzed for its content of GLA by an independent laboratory—one other than the manufacturer.

17. *Is there any remedy that can help smokers?*
Of course, the best way for smokers to help themselves (and others) is to stop smoking! But *antioxidant vitamins will help reduce the stress of the poisons of nicotine and tar on the body—lots of vitamins C and E and beta carotene.* Research has shown that the amino acid cysteine helps prevent damage by alcohol and certain chemicals. The chemicals studied involved in cigarette smoking were acetaldehyde and cadmium, a heavy metal. In light of such evidence, smokers and the nonsmokers that surround them might find it beneficial to take cysteine. Cysteine itself is prone to oxidation and is not efficient in the body, and neither is its alternate form L-cysteine, which is most often found commercially. So look for the protected form of cysteine, known as N-acetyl cysteine. This amino acid is protected from oxidation, helping it to be assimilated by cells.

18. *Is it better to eat fresh herbs or dried herbs?*
Eating freshly picked herbs will ensure that you receive all of the active ingredients contained in the herb. However, to get the same amount of active ingredients from a fresh herb as from its

dried, encapsulated alternative requires that you eat a huge amount of the fresh herb—often up to four pounds. So dried, preferably lyophilized herb capsules are your best bet. The fresh herb does contribute one thing that the dry herb does not: water. The water contained within the fresh herb is a natural vehicle that magnifies the action of the dispersed active principles. *If you eat fresh herbs regularly, not as condiments but as main food sources, there is no need to take herb capsules.*

19. *I've heard that B₁₂ can treat mental illnesses like Alzheimer's disease. Is this true?*

You are probably referring to a study conducted in the Netherlands that gained some notoriety a few years ago and was published in the *Journal of Orthomolecular Psychiatry*. In this study, doctors tested patients with Alzheimer's, as well as those with brain disorders related to alcohol abuse. They found that all patients had low levels of B_{12} and zinc and concluded that therapeutic doses of B_{12} and zinc can prevent this type of irreversible brain damage. Although B_{12} deficiency has been linked to different psychiatric conditions, the evidence is not conclusive that B_{12} can reverse brain damage due to Alzheimer's disease.

20. *What are bromelins?*

Bromelins are natural enzymes found in pineapple that digest protein, up to 900 times their weight. They have been used in the treatment of pancreatic insufficiency, as a substitute for enzymes released by the pancreas that digest protein, as well as in weight control, to reduce cholesterol, for elimination of deposits in such conditions as cellulitis, and as a diuretic for the regulation of fluids. *Bromelins are commonly used to relieve the sensation of bloating after large meals including a great deal of meat.* They are taken in tablet form. Fresh pineapple contains bromelins, but these enzymes tend to break down during the drying and processing of candied or dried pineapple chunks.

21. *Does drinking a lot of water wash away minerals?*

No. The body regulates the intake of minerals from the foods or supplements we take in, and water has little to do with the absorption process. Water may even help the process by providing a vehicle for dissemination of minerals in solution.

FOR FURTHER READING

Anderson, R. "Ascorvate-mediated Stimulation of Neutrophil Motility and Lymphocyte Transformation by Inhibition of the Peroxidase/Peroxide/Halide System in Vitro and in Vivo." *American Journal of Clinical Nutrition* 34 (1981).

Anderson, R. "Assessment of Oral Ascorbate in Three Children with Chronic Granulomatous Disease and Defective Neutrophil Motility over a 2-Year Period." *Clinical and Experimental Immunology* 43 (1981).

Bray, G., ed. *Recent Advances in Obesity Research.* London: John Libbey and Co., 1978.

Cheng, H. H., et al. "The Anti-tumor Effect of Cultivated *Ganoderma lucidum* Extract." *Journal of the Chinese Oncology Society* 1 (1982).

Cheraskin, E.; Ringsdorf, W.; and Medford, F. "The Ideal Daily Vitamin A Intake." *International Journal of Vitamin and Nutrition Research* 46 (1976).

Clegg, R. J.; Middleton, B.; Bell, G. D.; and White, D. A. "Inhibition of Hepatic Cholesterol Synthesis by Monoterpenes Administered in Vivo." *Biochemical Pharmacology* 29 (1980).

Cureton, Thomas. *The Physiological Effects of Wheat Germ Oil on Humans in Exercise.* Springfield, Ill.: Charles C. Thomas, 1972.

Day, Charles. "Sitosterol: Nature's Natural Cholesterol Neutralizer." *Nutrition & Dietary Consultant* (June 1985).

Foley, D. "Natural Sparks to Get Your Energy Sizzling." *Prevention* (February 1985).

Fredericks, Carlton. *Eat Well, Get Well, Stay Well.* New York: Grosset and Dunlap, 1980.

Fredericks, Carlton. *New and Complete Nutrition Handbook.* Canoga Park, Calif.: Major Books, 1976.

Hoppe, H. A.; Levring, T.; and Tanaka, Y., eds. *Marine Algae in Pharmaceutical Science.* Berlin: Walter de Gruyter, 1979.

Kirschmann, J., and Dunne, L. *Nutrition Almanac.* New York: McGraw-Hill, 1984.

Leibovitz, B. "The Effects of Marine Fish Oils on Health and Disease." *Nutrition Update* 5 (1986).

Littaru, G.; Ho, L.; and Folkers, K. "Deficiency of Coenzyme Q_{10} in Human Heart Disease. Parts 1 and 2. *International Journal for Vitamin and Nutrition Research* 42 (1972).

Mathews-Roth, M. "Antitumour Activity of Beta-Carotene, Canthaxanthin, and Phytoene." *Oncology* 39 (1982).

McAleer, Neil. *The Body Almanac.* New York: Doubleday, 1985.

Nestel, P. et al. "Suppression by Diets Rich in Fish Oil of Very Low Density Lipoprotein Production in Man." *Journal of Clinical Investigation* 74 (1984).

Phillipson, B. et al. "Reduction of Plasma Lipids, Lipoproteins, and Apoproteins by Dietary Fish Oils in Patients with Hypertriglyceridemia." *New England Journal of Medicine* 312 (1985).

Serrentino, J. *All about Vitamins.* Technical manual. Montreal: Bioforce, 1989.

Shin, H. W. et al. "Studies on Inorganic Composition and Immunopotentiating Activity of *Ganoderma lucidum* in Korea." *Korean Journal of Pharmacology* 16 (1985).

Sprince, H.; Parker, G.; and Smith, G. "Comparison of Protection by L-Ascorbic acid, L-Cysteine, and Adrenergic-blocking Agents against Acetaldehyde, Acrolein, and formaldehyde Toxicity: Implications in Smoking." *Agents and Actions* 9 (1979).

Von Schacky, C.; Fischer, S.; and Weber, P. "Long-Term Effects of Dietary Marine r-3 Fatty acids upon Plasma and Cellular Function, and Eicosanoid Formation in Humans." *Journal of Clinical Investigation* 76 (1985).

Glossary

Active principles: The ingredients extracted from a plant that have therapeutic qualities.

Adjuvant therapy: Therapy which may be either a remedy or a treatment program that supports and enhances the action of another treatment or remedy.

Aldehyde: A colorless, volatile liquid with a suffocating smell obtained by oxidation of the alcohol, acetaldehyde.

Alkaloid: One of a large group of organic base substances found in plants, usually very bitter and some of them very poisonous.

Allergen: A substance that causes an allergic reaction.

Allopathic medicine: Treatment of disease by inducing an opposite condition to the disease itself. Allopathic medicine underlies the conventional use of drugs in Western medicine.

Ames test: A test for mutagens involving innoculation of a strain of bacteria, *salmonella typhimurium*, with the suspected substance.

Amino acid: General name for any of 80 naturally occuring organic acids incorporating one or more amino groups. Twenty of them are the building blocks of protein.

AN/TN: A way of determining the quality of an amino acid product by measuring the nitrogen balance.

Analgesic: Having a pain killing effect.

Anthelmintic: Expelling or destroying parasitic worms, especially in the intestine.

Antibacterial: Killing bacteria.

Anticoagulant: Hindering clotting of the blood.

Antigen: A substance that stimulates the body to produce antibodies.

Antioxidant: Preventing reactions with oxygen and the formation of free radicals. Antioxidants are useful as preservatives and in combatting disease.

Antiphlogistic: Reducing inflammation.

Antispasmodic: Preventing constriction of the muscles.

Antiviral: Killing viruses.

Astringent: Causing contraction of the skin and the soft tissues of the body.

Aromatherapy: The therapeutic use of essential oils by application to the skin, ingestion, and inhalation.

Arteriosclerosis: A chronic disease of the arteries characterized by abnormal thickening, stiffening, and loss of elasticity of aterial walls through fatty deposits in the blood.

Avogadro's number: 6.023×10^{23}, the number of particles, real or imagined, of the type specified by the chemical formula of a substance in one gram mole of the substance.

Bactericidal: Killing bacteria.

BCAA: A branch-chained amino acid used as a fuel pack for athletes.

Bio-assay: Determination of the potency of a substance by testing its effect on a living organism or *in vitro* as compared with the effect of a standard preparation or substance.

Bioenergetics: The study of energy transformation in all living beings.

Bioflavonoid: A generic term for a group of compounds that are widely distributed in plants and that are concerned with the maintenance of a normal state of the walls of small blood vessels.

Biological products: Products comprised of organic elements that yield a compatable energy pattern with ills of the body and make the product biologically active.

Bionosode: A remedy of low potency consisting of a biological substance that emulates the pathological effects of a disease at a specific site in the body, such as an organ.

Biphasic effect: The two-stage effect of a substance on the body, phase one being the action of the substance on the body, and phase two, the body's reaction to the substance. This is typical of allopathic treatment.

Bouillon: A decoction that uses the whole plant and is drunk like a soup.

Certified biological: A guarantee that a product has been tested for contaminants and is distilled from organically grown plants.

Chelation: The chemical process by which a single mineral is bound to an amino acid and is thus more easily metabolized.

Ch'i: In Chinese medicine, a cardinal energy of the body that flows normally, without interruption along meridians in a healthy person.

Chromotographic machine: A device that determines the active ingredients of a particular substance by generating bands of colour on a photographic plate.

Chronic condition: A recurring ailment caused by an altered biological state.

Cholesterol: A substance widely distributed in animal tissue important in metabolism. High levels of cholesterol in the blood can lead to heart disease.

Decoction: A tea made by placing plant or plant parts in cold water and bringing them to a boil.

DIN: A drug identification number assigned by the US Food and Drug Administration or by Health and Welfare Canada. Under DIN regulations, therapeutic applications of natural products cannot be named on the label.

Diuretic: Promoting excretion of urine.

DNA (dioxyribonucleic acid): A nucleic acid that stores genetic information in the body.

Drug picture: A way of cataloguing a homeopathic remedy according to its effects on a healthy person matched to diseases that produce the same effect.

Effector: A tissue, cell or gland which causes an organ or muscle to contract or secrete in direct response to nerve impulses.

Elixir: A distilled maceration of plant material in alcohol mixed with sugar, used to invigorate the body.

Endorphin: A morphine-like substance secreted by the pituitary gland that acts as a natural pain killer.

Entropy: A state of disorder caused by the ingestion of substances incompatable with the bio-energy of the body with a subsequent loss of health; a diminished capacity for spontaneous change as can happen with age.

Enzymes: Proteins that catalyze biochemical reactions.

Epinephrine: Adrenalin, a hormone secreted into the bloodstream by the adrenal gland.

Essential oil: That part of a plant's immune system extracted by vapor distillation as a fragrant, pure liquid. Natural oils are much stronger than synthetically-derived oils.

Esters: Any compound formed an alchohol and an acid by the removal of water.

Ethers: Compounds produced by the action of acids on alchohol, resulting in a colourless, volatile liquid.

Excipient: A non-medical substance such as coatings, bindings, and fillings used to manufacture tablets.

Expectorant: Promoting coughing or spitting.

Extract: A percolation in water or alchohol of powdered or chopped plant parts. *See also* Lixiviation.

Freeze-drying: The removal of water from frozen material by evaporation in a vacuum at a low temperature.

Free radicals: An atoms or molecule having at least one unpaired electron. When free radicals react with a radical (or stable compound) a free radical is produced which may become a chain reaction, producing damage to tissues in the body.

Fungicidal: Killing fungus growths.

Glucose: A form of sugar found in certain foods, especialy fruit, and in the blood that is a major source of energy.

Infusion: A tea made by pouring boiling water over plant parts.

Inhalation: A tea of aromatic plants placed in hot water so that the vapor may be inhaled.

Healing crisis: An initial worsening of an illness induced by a homeopathic remedy.

Histamine: A substance found in all body tissues that fulfills a number of functions, including dilation of the capillaries, contraction of muscles, promoting gastric se retion, and acceleration of the heart rate.

High-density lipoprotein (LDL): *See* Lipoproteins.

Holograph: A three-dimensional representation of an object produced by interference between a coherent beam of light (from a laser) and light diffracted from the same beam by the object.

Homeopathy: Treatment of disease by substances (usually in minute doses) that in healthy persons would produce symptoms like those of the disease.

Hydrolysate: A product of hydrolysis, in which a substance is decomposed into simpler compounds by reaction with water.

Hypertension: High blood pressure.

Hypothalamus: The gland that controls all other glands in the body.

Hypothermic: A condition in which the body temperature is lowered by constriction of the blood vessels.

High-density lipoproteins (HDL): *See* Lipoproteins.

International Units (IU): A quantity of a biological substance (vitamin, hormone, antibiotic, antitoxin) or its equivalent based on a bioassay that produces a particular biological effect agreed upon internationally.

Ketone: One of a class of organic compounds important in the synthesis of organic compounds.

Kirlean aura: A discharge of sparks produced by the electro-magnetic fields around the body. Disorders of the body produce changes in the Kirlean aura.

Krebs cycle: Cellular respiration, a cycle of chemical reactions that releases energy and allows the cell to fulfill its function in the biosystem.

Leukocyte: White blood cells or corpuscle responsible for combatting infection.

Leukotrienes: A group of compounds made from arachidonic acid by the enzyme lipoxygenase. They are chemical mediations in the allergy response, working as potent bronchoconstrictors.

Liniments: A combination of rubbing alchohol and a maceration of plant material to stimulate circulation of an injured or sore area of the body.

Lipids: Fats and fat-like substances (waxes and oils) that are insoluble in water. Cholesterol is a form of lipid.

Lipoproteins: Protein combined with a lipid. Lipoproteins found in the blood are classified as Low Density (LDL), Very Low Density (VLDL) and High Density (HDL). LDLs and VLDLs are composed of large amounts of cholesterol and at high levels are associated with hardening of the arteries and coronary heart disease.

Lixiviation: The separation of substances into soluble and insoluble constituents by percolation.

LMR (*Limite Maximale des Residus Nocifs*): The maximum amount of toxic residues permitted in herbs and other commercial products of a herbal nature as tested by independent laboratories in participating European countries.

Low-density lipoproteins (LDL): *See* Lipoprotein.

Lyophilization: *See* Freeze-drying.

Maceration: The process by which plants are chopped and soaked in alchohol, water, or wine.

Macrophage: An effector cell found in tissues that eats foreign cells such as bacteria and fungus.

Markers: That part of an active principle of a biological substance that contains a genetic "memory" of the organism from which it is extracted, permitting the substance to convey the full benefit of the organism. Synthetic substances do not have markers.

Meridian system: A basic concept of Chinese medicine which describes the body as having energy channels or meridians along which a cardinal energy, or ch'i, flows uninterruptedly in healthy persons.

Metabolism: The process by which nutritive material is changed into living matter and the transformation by which such energy is made available to living beings.

Mineral complex: Minerals produced by a Krebs cycle acid and thus more readily metabolized.

Mole: A unit of measurement of chemical quantities in which the mass is said to be numerically equal to the mass of the molecules it contains. *See also* Avogadro's number.

Monocyte: A large type of white corpuscle that eats larger particles invading the body such as bacteria and fungus.

Mother tincture: The original extract of a natural substance used as the basis for a homeopathic remedy.

Motoyama AMI machine: Apparatus for Measuring the Functions of the Meridians and the Internal Organs, a diagnostic device designed by Japanese researcher Hiroshi Motoyama that makes use of electrical information from acupuncture points.

Mucinolytic: Thinning mucus secretions.

Mutagen: A substance that produces damage to the genetic material known as DNA, causing cell death or cancerous changes.

Natural substance: A substance, such as sugar, that exists naturally and does not have to be synthesized, but which, as a result of refining or manufacturing processes, may not be pure.

Naturopathy: The treatment of a disease by seeking to promote natural recovery through the use of organic remedies, natural foods, and physical therapies such as massage.

Neurotoxic: Toxic or corrupting to the nervous system by the poisoning or destruction of nerves.

Neutrophil: A type of white blood cell that eats bacteria and small particles.

Neutrophil fatigue: A disorder of the nervous system characterised by subnormal activity of leukocytes.

Nutrients: Multi-vitamin complexes made from dehydrated supplements or specially processed whole foods.

Nucleic acids: Organic acids, the principle ones being DNA (deoxyribonucleic acid) and RNA (ribonucleic acid).

Organic: A substance derived from plants grown in unpolluted soil without harmful herbicides, insecticides, fertilizers, or fungicidals.

Oxidation: The chemical reaction that increases the oxygen content of a substance. Biologically, oxidation results in the release of energy in the body.

Peptide-bonded: A form of amino acid from plants and animals more easily metabolized by the body.

Phagocyte: A cell that has the ability to ingest and destroy foreign particles that invade the body, such as bacteria and dust.

Phenol: An organic compound derivative of an aromatic hyrdocarbon, especially benzene, used in dilution as an antiseptic and disinfectant.

Phytotherapy: The therapeutic use of plants.

Plasma: The liquid part of the blood; the viscous living matter that surround the nucleus of a cell.

Plasmolysis: A method of culturing yeast to make tonics.

Polypeptide: A molecule consisting of numerous amino acids linked together by peptide bonds.

Potentiation: The process of diluting homeopathic remedies in order to realize their effectiveness.

Poultice: The combination of a decoction with medicinal clay applied to the skin.

Protein Efficiency Ratio (PER): A way of ascertaining the quality of an amino acid product by measuring the weight gain of an animal fed the protein.

Recommended Dietary Allowance (RDA): The minimum daily dosage of a specific vitamin or mineral required to prevent deficiency.

Resonance: A biophysical phenomenum where the body is held to resonate at a given electro-magnetic frequency based on the oscillation of atoms. Disease or illness disrupts the resonant frequency.

Secretolytic: Increasing the secretion and liquifaction of mucus.

Sedative: Relaxing the body and muscles, inducing sleep.

Semi-synthetic vitamins: A synthetic vitamin that has been combined with nutrients or other vitamins from natural sources.

Serotonin: A substance found in the blood that constricts the blood vessels.

Sublingual: Under the tongue.

Standardized herbs: Plants which have been batch tested to determine safe levels of active principles.

Succussion: The mechanical shaking of a tincture diluted with water to produce a homeopathic remedy.

Synergy: The enhancement of one ingredient by the presence of another.

Synthetic: Manufactured in a laboratory and not normally produced in nature; may also be a copy of a natural substance.

Syrups: A combination of an infusion or maceration with refined or raw sugar, honey, or treacle, generally for coughs.

Terpenes: Any of a large number of hydrocarbons found in essential oils, especialy oranges and conifers.

Tincture: A maceration or percolation in alchohol of fresh plant material to extract a remedy.

Trace minerals: Minerals necessary for health that are present in the body in minute amounts.

Vapor distillation: A method of distilling plant parts in a still to yield an essential oil and a hydrolysate.

Viricidal: Killing viruses.

Voll machine: A diagnostic device invented by the German physician Reinhard Voll that makes use of electrical information from acupuncture points for the diagnosis of illness. The Voll machine can also be used to compare the energy pattern of a natural remedy against that of the body.

Wraps: Soaking of a sterile gauze bandage in a decoction to bandage an ailing limb.

Selected
Bibliography

Anderson, J., and Sieling, B. "High-Fiber Diets for Diabetics: Unconventional But Effective." *Geriatrics* 36 (1981).

Armstrong. D.; Sohal, R. S.; Cutler, R.; and Slater, T., eds. *Free Radicals in Molecular Biology, Aging and Disease.* New York: Raven Press, 1984.

Bach, E. *The Bach Flower Remedies.* New Canaan, Conn.: Keats Publishing Co., 1977.

Baerlein, E., and Dower, A. *Healing with Radionics: The Science of Healing Energy.* Wellingborough, England: Thorsons Publishers, 1980.

Barbeau, A.; Growdon, J. E.; and Whurtman, R. J. *Nutrition and the Brain.* New York: Raven Press, 1979.

Beiser, Arthur. *Physics.* Menlo Park, Calif.: Cummings Publishing Company, 1973.

Black, Dean. *Health at the Crossroads.* Springville, Utah: Tapestry Press, 1988.

Block, E. "The Chemistry of Garlic and Onions." *Scientific American* 252 (1985).

Burnet, Sir Macfarlane. "The Mechanism of Immunity." Readings from Scientific American: Immunology. San Francisco: W. H. Freeman and Company, 1976.

Cameron, E.; Pauling, L.; and Leibovitz, B. "Ascorbic Acid and Cancer: A Review." *Cancer Research* 39 (1979).

Cureton, Thomas. *The Physiological Effects of Wheat Germ Oil on Humans in Exercise.* Springfield, Ill.: Charles C. Thomas, 1972.

Curtis, Helena. *Biology.* New York: Worth Publishers, 1975.

Day, L., and de la Warr, G. *New Worlds beyond the Atom.* London: Vincent Stuart, 1966.

Dice, L. R. *Man's Nature and Nature's Man.* Ann Arbor: University of Michigan Press, 1955.

"Does Nature Know Best? Natural Carcinogens in American Food." A Report by the American Council on Science and Health. Revised. Reprinted July 1987.

Dubos, René. *Man Adapting.* New Haven and London: Yale University Press, 1980.

Dubos, René. *Mirage of Health: Utopias, Progress, and Biological Change.* New Brunswick and London: Rutgers University Press, 1987.

Facinelli, Paul. "A Repair Kit for Varicose Veins." *Prevention* (February 1985).

Fisher, Richard B. *A Dictionary of Body Chemistry.* London: Granada Publishing, 1983.

Foley, D. "Clean Out Your Cholesterol." *Prevention* (July 1985).

Fredericks, Carlton. *Psycho-Nutrition.* New York: Grosset and Dunlap, 1972.

Fudenberg, H. H.; Stites, D. P.; Caldwell, J. L.; and Wells, J. V., eds. *Basic and Clinical Immunology.* Los Altos, Calif.: Lange Medical Publications, 1976.

Garn, S. M. "Culture and the Direction of Human Evolution." *Human Biology* 35 (1963).

Gerber, Richard. *Vibrational Medicine.* Santa Fe: Bear and Co., 1988.

Grad, B. *New Frontiers in the Treatment of the Whole Person,* ed. Otto and Knight. Chicago: Nelson-Hall, 1979.

Hahnnemann, S. *Organon of Medicine.* Los Angeles: J. P. Tarcher, 1982.

Hallett, F. R.; Speight, P. A.; Stinson, R. H.; and Graham, W. G. *Introductory Biophysics.* Toronto: Methuen Publications, 1977.

Heaton, D., ed. *Dietary Fiber: Current Developments of Importance to Health.* London: John Libbey and Company, 1978.

Hoagland, H., and Burhoe, R. W. *Evolution and Man's Progress.* New York: Columbia University Press, 1962.

Ingelfinger, F. J. "Medicine: Meritorious or Meretricious?" *Science* 200 (1978).

Jensen, Bernard. "Chlorella: The Jewel of the East." *The Vitamin Supplement* (May 1988).

Kinderleherer, J. "What to Eat When You're Sick." *Prevention* (September 1985).

Kirschmann, J. D., and Dunne, L. J. *Nutrition Almanac*. New York: McGraw-Hill, 1984.

Kushi, Michio. *How to See Your Health: Book of Oriental Diagnosis*. Tokyo: Japan Publications, 1980.

Leibovitz, B. "The Effects of Marine Fish Oils on Health and Disease." *Nutrition Update* 5 (1986).

Leibovitz, Brian. "Nutrition and Allergy." *Nutrition Update*, Vol. 1, no. 7 (1986).

Lorenzi, G., and Cogoli, A. "Effect of Plasmolyzed Yeast Preparations on Cellular Functions." *Swiss Biotech* 3 (1985).

Luce, G. *Biological Rhythms in Human and Animal Physiology*. New York: Dover Publications, 1971.

Machlin, L. J., and Bendich, A. "Free Radical Tissue Damage: Protective Role of Antioxidant Nutrients." *Federation of American Societies for Experimental Biology Journal* 1 (1987).

Maleskey, G. "Thin Your Blood and Live Longer." *Prevention* (May 1987).

Matthews, D. M., and Laster, L. "Absorption of Protein Digestion Products: A Review." *Gut* 6 (1966).

McAleer, Neil. *The Body Almanac*. New York: Doubleday and Company, 1985.

McGilvery, R. W. *Biochemistry: A Functional Approach*. Philadelphia, London, and Toronto: W. B. Saunders Company, 1970.

Morrison, R. T., and Boyd, R. N. *Organic Chemistry*. Boston: Allyn and Bacon, 1973.

Motoyama, H., and Brown, R. *Science and the Evolution of Consciousness*. Brookline, Mass.: Autumn Press, 1978.

National Academy of Sciences. *The Health Effects of Nitrate, Nitrite, and N-Nitroso Compounds*. Washington, D.C.: National Academy Press, 1981.

Peto, R. *Assessment of Risk from Low Level Exposure to Radiation and Chemicals*. New York: Plenum Press, 1985.

Phillips M., and Baetz, A., eds. *Diet and Resistance to Disease*. New York: Plenum Press, 1981.

Philpott, W. H. *Brain Allergies: The Psycho-Nutrient Connection*, New Canaan, Conn.: Keats Publishing, 1980.

Polanyi, M. *The Study of Man*. Chicago: University of Chicago Press, 1959.

Porcellati, G.; Amaducci, C.; and Gallo, C. *Function and Metabolism of Phospholipids.* New York: Plenum Press, 1976.

Prasad, A. S., and Oberleas, D., eds. *Trace Elements in Human Health and Disease.* New York: Academic Press, 1976.

Pryor, W., ed. *Free Radicals in Biology.* Vol. VI. Orlando, Fla.; Academic Press, 1984.

Rao, C. *The Chemistry of Lignins.* Walthair, India: Andhra University Press, 1978.

Robertson, M. "Nerves, Molecules and Embryos." *Nature* 278 (April 26, 1979).

Rubin, H. "Cancer As a Dynamic Developmental Disorder." *Cancer Research* 45 (July 1985).

Sacks, Oliver. *A Leg to Stand On.* New York: Harper and Row, 1984.

Searles, H. *The Nonhuman Environment.* New York: International University Press, 1960.

Selye, H. *The Stress of Life.* New York: McGraw-Hill, 1976.

Shamberger, R. *Nutrition and Cancer.* New York: Plenum Press, 1984.

Sies, Helmut, ed. *Oxidative Stress.* Orlando, Fla.: Academic Press, 1985.

Stich, H. F. *Carcinogens and Mutagens in the Environment.* Boca Raton, Fla.: CRC Press, 1982.

Tansley, D. *Radionics and the Subtle Anatomy of Man.* Essex, England: Health Science Press, 1972.

Trowell, H.; Burkitt, D.; and Heaton, K., eds. *Dietary Fiber, Fiber-Depleted Foods and Disease.* London: Academic Press, 1985.

Vahouny, G., and Kritchevsky, D., eds. *Dietary Fiber: Basic and Clinical Aspects.* New York: Plenum Press, 1986.

Vaugn, L. "Stopping the Pain of Migraine." *Prevention* (July 1985).

Wacker, A., and Hilbig, W. "Virus-Inhibition by *Echinacea purpurea.*" *Planta Med* 33 (1978).

Weiner, M. A. *Earth Medicine.* New York: Macmillan, 1980.

Weiner, M. A. "Herbs and Immunity." *The Herbal Healthline* 1 (1989).

Weymouth, L. "The Electrical Connection." *New York Magazine* (November 24, 1980).

Wurtman, R., and Wurtman, J. "Carbohydrates and Depression." *Scientific American* (January 1989).

Zarrow, Susan. "Keep Your Eyes Young and Sharp." *Prevention* (March 1985).

Holistic Health Associations and Resources

American Association of Naturopathic Physicians
P.O. Box 2579
Kirkland, WA
98083
206-27-6034

American Holistic Medical Association
2002 Eastlake Avenue, E.
Seattle, WA
98102
206-322-6842

Canadian Holistic Healing Association
1965 West Broadway
Vancouver, BC
V6J 1Z3

Canadian Holistic Medical Association
700 Bay Street
Suite 604
P.O. Box 101
Toronto, ON
M5G 1Z6
416-599-0447

International Association of Holistic Health Practitioners
3419 Thom Blvd.
Las Vegas, Nevada
89130
702-873-4542

International Academy of Nutrition and Preventive Medicine
P.O. Box 5832
Lincoln, NE
68505
402-467-2716

International Foundation For Homeopathy
2366 Eastlake Avenue E.
Suite 301
Seattle, WA
98102
206-324-8230

Nutrition Education Association
3647 Glen Haven
Houston, TX
77025
713-665-2946

Quebec Medical Holistic Association
P.O. Box 478
Cookshire, PQ
J0R 1M0
819-875-3565

Index

Anti-flatulents, 181
Antigens, 47
Anti-inflammatories, 82, 87, 182, 203
Anti-oxidants, 38, 108, 132, 136, 165–166, 187 189, 206. *See also* Vitamins; Free radicals
Antihistamines, 178
Antiseptics, 95, 184. *See also* Disinfectants
Antispasmodics, 71, 72, 87, 89, 90, 176, 179
Anthelmintics, 72 86, 90
Anxiety. *See* Anti-depressants
Appetite. *See* Digestion
Arginine, 175–176
Arnica (*Arnica montana*), 102
Aromatherapy, 63–64
Arthritis and rheumatism, 53, 131, 185, 189, 190, 203, 209
Artichoke (*Cynara scolymus*), 111, 183
Ascorbic acid. *See* Vitamin C
Asthma, 211
Astragalus (Qiang gan ruan jian tang), 206–207
Astringents, 71, 181
Atheriosclerosis, 136
Athlete's foot, 82
Autoimmune diseases, 189–90. *See also* Arthritis and rheumatism
Avogadro's number, 49
B-factor, 174
Bach, Dr. Edward, 54
Bactericidals. *See* Anti-bacterials
Balsam fir (*Abies balsamia*), 104
Baptisia leucantha (Wild or False Indigo), 174
Batch testing, 31–32, 110
Baths and washes, healing, 83
Bay leaves (*Laurus nobilis*), 74, 89
Bearberry (*Arctostaphylos uva-ursi*), 118
Beta-carotene, 107, 167, 168, 171, 206, 208. *See also* Vitamin A
Binders, 42

Bio-assay, 31–32
Biochemical balance, 7–8
Bioenergetics, 4–7
Bioflavonoids, 108, 188, 194
Biological product, 13–14
Biological remedies, 23
Bionosodes, 54–55
Biotin, 131
Biphasic effect, 129
Birch, tap (*Betula alba*), 104, 184
Blood
    pressure, high, 72, 83–84, 85, 104, 123, 155, 188
    purifiers, 83–84, 104, 184
Boils, 103
Bouillons, 101
Brain stimulants, 89, 90, 156
Branch-chain amino acids (BCAA), 40, 139
Breast pain, 102
Breath, shortness of, 104
Brewer's yeast, 143
Bromelins, 213
Bronchitis, 101
Bryonia (Bryonia dioica), 174
Buckthorn (*Rhamnus cathartica*), 117–118, 180, 181
Burns, 82
Butterbur, (*Petasites hybridus*), 185
Cactus, 117
Caffeine, 211
Calcium, 131, 133, 188, 194
Camphor, 117
Cancer, 79, 135–136, 165, 167, 190–195, 203, 207
    and vitamins, 135–136. *See also* Carcinogens
Capsules, 41–44, 125–126, 140, 172
Carcinogens, 107–109, 136
Carrot, Wild (*Daucus carota*), 88–89
Catalase, 165–166
Cataracts, 131, 136
Cayenne, 176
Cedar, essential oils of, 70
Cellular respiration, 120

231 ∎

Elixirs, 104–105
Emotions, and illness, 53–55
Emphysema, 131
Energy patterns, 3–7, 11, 13, 50–53, 98
English Ivy (*Hederis helix*), 176
Entropy, 8, 122. *See also* Thermodynamics
Enzymes, 119–120, 155–156, 157. *See also* Coenzymes; Coenzyme Q10
EPA. *See* Eicosapentenoic acid
Ephedra (*Ephedra Sinica*), 177
Epinephrine, 53
Essential oils, 2–3, 14, 35–37, 59, 63–91, 96, 97, 99
   of bay leaf, 74
   of carrot, wild, 88–89
   of cedar bark, 70,
   of chamomile, 74, 87, 186
   of cloves, 73, 86
   of evening primrose, 32, 211–212
   of garlic, 194
   of goldenrod, 174
   of juniper, 184
   of lavender, 69, 79, 81–83, 177
   of marjoram, 87–88
   of melissa, 178
   of mint, 90
   of orange, 194
      leaves, 74
      peel, 80
   of rosemary, 67–68, 83–86
   of verbena, 67
   of sandalwood, 78
Esters, 72
Ethers, 71
Eucalyptus
   (*Eucalyptus radiata*), 103
   (*Eucalytpus globulus*), 102. *See also* Teas
Eugenol, 73
Evening primrose (*Oenothera biennis*), 32, 211–212
Excipients, 42, 115–116

Exercise,
   mental, 24–25
   spiritual, 25
Expectorant, 81, 89, 176
"Extra Virgin" oils, 38
Extraction of oils, cold-pressed, 37–38
Extracts, 14–15
   of artichoke, 111, 183
   of aloe vera, 211
   of baptisia, 174
   of birch, 184
   of butterbur, 185
   of chlorella, 173
   of echinacea, 105, 174
   of ephedra, 177
   of glandular tissue, 179
   of hops, 178
   of horse chestnut, 186
   of melissa, 178
   of oat, 174
   of orange peel, 79
   of passion flower, 178
   of potentilla, 181
   of reishi mushroom, 207
   of restharrow, 184
   of shiitake mushroom, 207
Eye problems, 131, 188, 189
False Solomon's seal (*Smilacina racemosa*), 103
Fat soluble vitamins. *See* Vitamins
Fatigue, 89, 90, 157, 174
Fennel (*Foeniculum vulgare*), 180–181
Fever, 87, 89, 174
Fiber, 181, 188, 204
Fillers, 42
Fish oils, 123, 203–204
Flavonoids, 96, 116
Flu, 21, 104, 174–175
Food allergy. *See* Allergy
Food and Drug Administration. *See* Regulation
Food additives, 135–136
Food intolerance, 134

Hyperactivity, remedies for, 211
Hypertension. *See* Blood pressure
Hyperthermics, 72
Hypothermics, 70, 72
Illness and personality, 55
Immune
  stimulants, 71, 79, 89, 105, 174
  system, 53, 79, 191, 206–207
Infection, 85, 86, 90
Infusions, 101. *See also* Teas
Inhalations, 77, 81, 102
Inorganic chemicals, 14
Inositol, 131, 155
Insomnia, 178
Interferon, 206, 207
International units, 121
Interro diagnostic machine, 51
Iodine, 131
Ipecac, 176
Irish moss, 78
Iron, 131, 167
Ischemia, 136
Isoleucine. *See* Amino acids
IU. *See* International units
Ivy. *See* English ivy
Juniper (*Juniperus communis*), 104,
  184
Ketones, 72–73
Kidney problems, 84, 136, 184–185,
  201
Kirlian auras, 51
Knotweed (*Polygonum aviculare*),
  182, 184
Krebs cycle, 143
L-glutathione peroxidase. *See*
  Glutathione
Labels
  and batch-testing, 32
  in Europe, 36
  of amino acids, 138
  of essential oils, 2–3, 36, 69, 75,
    82, 84
  of glandular extracts, 210
  of homeopathic remedies, 55
  of tinctures, 114

of vitamins, 121, 127, 129, 130,
  132.
  See also Regulation
Lactic acid, 24, 41, 143
Lactose, 49
Larrea mexicana, 46
Lavender, 79
  spike (*Lavendula spica*), 81–82
  true (*Lavendula vera*), 69, 82–83,
    101, 177
Laxatives. *See* Constipation
LDL. *See* Low-density lipoproteins
Lecithin, 9–10, 45, 132, 205, 206
Lentinan, 207
Leucine. *See* Amino acids
Leukotrienes, 134
Limité Maximale di Résidue Nocifs,
  12
Liniments, 103
Lipid peroxidation, 164
Lipofuscin, 164
Liquid health products, 44–45
Liquid vitamins. *See* Vitamins
Liver problems, 83, 84, 107, 172,
  181, 182, 183
Lixiviation, 105, 115
LMR. *See* Limité Maximale di
  Résidue Nocifs
Loosestrife (*Lythrum salicaria*), 181
Low-density lipoproteins (LDL),
  158, 203
Lubricants, 42
Lyophilization, 38–39, 99–100
Maceration, 14–15, 101–102.   *See
  also* Teas; Elixirs
Macrobiotic diet, 58
Magnesium, 131, 133
Mammary tumours, 79. *See also* Can-
  cer
Manganese, 167, 188, 190
Manufacturing, 31–45, 97–100,
  114. *See also* Regulations
Marjoram (*Origanum majorana*),
  87–88
Massage oil, 85

Pantothenic acid. *See* Vitamin B5
Paprika, 176
Passionflower (*Passiflora incarnata*), 178
Para-aminobenzoic acid, 157
Parasites, 86
PCBs. *See* Polychlorinated biphenyls
Peppermint (*Mentha piperita*), 90, 103
Peptide-bonded amino acids, 39–40, 138
PER. *See* Protein Efficiency Ratio
Personality type, and illness, 55
Peruvian bark (*Cinchona succirubra*), 183
Pesticides. *See* Toxins
Phenols, 72
Phenothiazine, 160
Phosphorus, 131, 188
Photosynthesis, 94
Phytotherapy, 61
Pine, juice of, 176
Plasmolysis, 33–35. *See also* Yeast
Pollutants, 120, 125, 135–136, 166
Poplar (*Populus tremula* spp.), 179
Poppy, 95
Potassium, 133, 188
Potentization, 49
Potentilla (*Potentilla tormentilla* spp.), 181
Poultices, 96, 102
Powders, 103, 142
Pre-menstrual syndrome. *See* menstruation
Preservatives, 84
Procarcinogens, 191
Prostaglandins, 211
Prostate problems, 179–180
Proteins, 188. *See also* amino acids
Protein Efficiency Ratio (PER), 138
Pro-vitamin A, 203
Purple boneset (*Eupatorium purpureum*), 103
Purple coneflower (*Echinacea purpurea*), 62, 174, 206
Pyroxidine. *See* Vitamin B6

Quercitin, 108, 109
Quinine, 95
Radiation injury, 136
Radicals, free. *See* Free radicals
RDA. *See* Ribonucleic acid
Recommended dietary allowances, 121–124, 207–208
Red clover (*Trifolium pratense*), 104–105
Refining, 38
Refrigeration, 120
Regulation, 124
   of labelling, 1–3, 12, 121
   of manufacturing,
      in Europe, 12
      in USA & Canada, 12–13
Reishi mushroom. *See* mushrooms
Remedies. *See* individual conditions
   (e.g., Aging, Flu, Surgery). *See also* Allopathic; Holism; Homeopathic; Naturopathic; Tonics; Immune system stimulants
Repellents, 79
Resonant frequency, 6
Respiratory problems, 174
Restharrow (*Ononis spinosa*), 184
Retinol, 167 *See also* Vitamin A
Rheumatism. *See* Arthritis and rheumatism
Ribonucleic acid, 131
Rice-bran oil, 132
Rosemary true (*Rosmarinus officinalis*), 67, 68, 83–84, 103, 104
   cultivated, 84–85
   Mediterranean, 85–86
S Transferase, 165,166
Sabal (*Sabal serratata*), 179
Safflower oil, 78
Saffron oil, 78
Sage,
   common garden (*Salvia officinalis*), 2
   sclarated (*Salvia sclaria*), 2
Salicin, 130
Saps, 104
Schizophrenia, 157

IBS: A Doctor's Plan For Chronic Digestive Troubles
by Dr Gerard Guillory   224 pages

The definitive, comprehensive easy-to-use preventive guide for the one in five people suffering from recurrent digestive problems.

$11.95 PB (US) $14.95 PB (CANADA)

CHINESE MASSAGE
A handbook of therapeutic massage
by Anhui Medical School and A.Lade   264 pages

Detailed massage instructions, showing ways to restore health and strengthen the body's defenses.

$12.95 PB (US) $15.95 PB (CANADA)

THE CHINESE EXERCISE BOOK
From ancient & modern China – exercises for well-being and the treatment of Illnesses
by Dahong Zhuo, MD   200 pages

Illustrated exercises both for preventive health and rehabilitation, including special programs for older and sedentary people.

$9.95 PB (US) $10.95 PB (CANADA)

SKILLS FOR SIMPLE LIVING
How-to Letters From the Home Front for Tomorrow's World
Edited by Betty Tillotson   192 pages

A thousand environmentally conscious household tips and designs from magazine letters from people with real-life experience.

$12.95 PB (US) $15.95 PB (CANADA)

THE CRAFT OF THE COUNTRY COOK
From A-Z: Over 1,000 Recipes and Food Ideas

730 pages

A unique encyclopedia of recipes, ingredients, processes, and creative ideas from *Countryside* magazines's food columnist.

$19.95 PB (US) $24.95 PB (CANADA)

For a free catalog of all our books, write to:

Hartley & Marks, Inc.   or to   Hartley & Marks, Ltd.
Post Office Box 147   3663 West Broadway
Point Roberts, WA   Vancouver, B.C.
98281   V6R 2B8
U.S.A   CANADA